99 Things You Wish

You Knew Before®…

Losing Fat 4 Life

A guide to taking charge of your
life and health

Brad King, M.S, MFS

www.99-series.com

The 99 Series
600 Brunet
Montreal, QC H4M1X8
Canada
323-203-0548

Disclaimer
The advice and strategies contained herein may not be suitable for every
individual. It is very important for anyone reading this book to consult a
doctor before making any changes in diet and lifestyle, or before taking
vitamin and/or food/beverage supplements. While all care is taken with the
accuracy of the facts and procedures in this book, the author accepts
neither liability nor responsibility to any person with respect to loss, injury or
damage caused, or alleged to be caused directly or indirectly, by the
information contained in this book. The purpose of this book is solely to
educate and inform. For medical advice, you should seek the individual,
personal advice and services of a medical professional.

First published by The 99 Series 2010

Cover designed and Layout by
Ginger Marks
DocUmeantDesigns
www.DocUmeantDesigns.com

Jennifer Kennedy Paine,
Developmental Editor

Distributed by DocUmeant Publishing

For inquiries about volume orders, please contact:

Helen Georgaklis
99 Book Series, Inc.
600 Brunet Avenue E
Montreal, Quebec
Canada
H4M 1X8

Helen@99-series.com

Printed in Canada
ISBN-13: 978-0-9866629-2-8 9.99 (paperback)
ISBN-10: 0986662925

WORDS OF PRAISE

FOR...

---

99 Things You Wish You Knew Before... Losing Fat 4 Life ®

"I want to share with you one of the most inspiring health researchers I have ever met. Brad King empowers individuals to understand how your body works in laymen terms. Brad will teach you how YOU can make your body healthy, how YOU can live the life you wanted to live." **−Dr. John Gray, *Author of Men are from Mars Women are from Venus***

"*Brad King is the "king" of fitness. His latest book delivers the no-nonsense quick fixes that will not only make you 'fit' 4 life but will also give you the vitality and stamina to keep off the pounds forever. I wish everybody had a Brad King in their corner.*" −**Ann Louise Gittleman, PhD, CNS,** *author of Zapped, Why Your Cell Phone Shouldn't be Your Alarm Clock and 1,268 Ways to Outsmart the Hazards of Electronic Pollution (HarperONE, 2010)*

"*Brad takes a challenging and often misunderstood subject and breaks it down into an easy-to-understand, easy-to-implement formula, one WITHOUT dieting. Anyone who has ever struggled with weight loss would be crazy to ignore the eye-opening information in this book. From the body to the mind – 'Losing Fat 4 Life' holds the answer you've been waiting for!*" −**Brenda Wade, PhD,** *Relationship Expert for CNN, NBC's Today Show*

DEDICATION

This book is dedicated to the thousands of individuals who have been confused and frustrated too many times to count in their quest to lose excess body fat for life.

May this book give you the answers you so desperately crave!

CONTENTS

ABOUT THE 99

SERIES

The 99 Series is a collection of quick, easy-to-understand guides that spell it all out for you in the simplest format; 99 points, one lesson per page. The book series is the one-stop shop for all readers tired of looking all over for self-help books. The 99 Series brings it all to you under one umbrella! The bullet point format that is the basis for all the 99 Series books was created purposely for today's fast-paced society. Not only does information have to be at our finger tips... we need it quickly and accurately without having to do much research to find it. But don't be fooled by the easy-to-read format. Each of the books in the series contains very thorough discussions from our roster of professional authors so that all the information you need to know is compiled into one book!

We hope that you will enjoy this book as well as the rest of the series. If you've enjoyed our books, tell your friends. And if you feel we need to improve something, please feel free to give us your feedback at www.99-series.com.

Helen Georgaklis
Founder & CEO, 99 Series

INTRODUCTION

Let me begin by congratulating you on the start of your **99 Things You Wish You Knew Before Losing Fat 4 Life** journey. The fact that you are beginning to read this book tells me that you are interested in one of the following areas:

- You've been carrying around a great deal of excess weight for as long as you can remember, and you are sick and tired (literally) of what it is doing to you, both physically and emotionally.
- You have a few extra pounds to lose and you would desperately love to find a way to get rid of them to fit into your old pair of jeans.

- You just want to enhance your health profile and experience more energy and vitality.

Regardless of why you are reading this book, or deciding to begin yet another diet (don't do it until you finish reading this book), the fact remains that you are interested in becoming a healthier individual no matter where you presently are in your life. The good news is that the principles that comprise the **99 Things You Wish You Knew Before Losing Fat 4 Life** are proven to help you look, feel, and perform your best. In other words, if you are willing to make a commitment to yourself and follow the information within this book, you can't help but create a more fulfilling life for yourself and those around you.

Believe it or not, your body was not designed to be fat. Until you realize that the great majority of the excess body fat you are presently living with is caused by the less than optimal choices you make (and have made) each day (and I'm not solely referring to your diet here) you will never be 100 percent successful at creating a healthy metabolism conducive to continual fat loss.

The truth is that your metabolism is tightly controlled by your choices of food, lifestyle (are you active or sedentary?), and environment (both internal and external). If you decide to place high-calorie, high-carb, and nutrient-void foods in your mouth each day or at least the great majority of the time, all the while living a sedentary existence with a constant mindset that basically says, "I'll never be lean, healthy, and energetic no matter what I do," guess what you can expect: A fat laden body with very little energy to speak of—other than when you borrow some energy from your very own system by relying on "Java" to get you through each day. Sound familiar? Unfortunately, most would say yes!

In order to turn your metabolism around and have it work FOR YOU instead of

AGAINST YOU, you need to learn how to stimulate the right amount of metabolism boosting signals. The principles you are about to learn in **99 Things You Wish You Knew Before Losing Fat 4 Life**, in combination with proper exercise (as outlined in the Exercise chapter) is designed to show you how to correct the problems associated with a dysfunctional metabolism and instead experience a metabolism that uses your very own fat reserves as a constant fuel source—24 hours each day, seven days a week.

This is in no way another diet program. In fact, it is just the opposite. Over the past ten years, I have used these exact same principles to help thousands of people around the globe change their lives by losing excess body fat and experiencing unlimited energy levels.

With the information in **99 Things You Wish You Knew Before Losing Fat 4 Life**, you will never have to count another calorie or go hungry again! In fact, you will learn that when the right food is consumed at the right intervals, combined with the right supplementation, food is actually your friend. I have never believed in dieting and have always known that fad diets are nothing more than a short-term solution to a lifelong problem—the inability to permanently lose excess body fat 24/7.

I guarantee you that after reading this book and applying its information, you will be saying hello to the NEW YOU before you know it!

Don't put off the life you deserve for one more minute. Jump in with both feet and an unwavering desire to make your dreams of becoming the healthiest you a reality! I

know you can do it this time; the question
is, are *you* ready to make it happen?

Yours in Abundant Health,

Brad King

CHAPTER 1

HOW DID WE GET THIS WAY—EVER EXPANDING WAIST LINES

According to experts in the area of early human nutrition, 99.99 percent of our genetic codes were formed before the advent of agriculture, approximately 10,000 years ago. What this means according to Dr. Boyd Eaton, a medical anthropologist at Emory University, Atlanta, is "nearly all of our biochemistry and physiology are fine-tuned to conditions of life that existed before 10,000 years ago. Genetically, our bodies are now virtually the same as they were then." The problem is our diet is not.

More and more members of the scientific community believe in a concept called, "fetal programming," which suggests that while still in the womb, a fetus can adapt genetically to various environmental cues. These cues, whether positive (as in drinking enough water, eating healthy foods, exercising, getting plenty of rest, and stressing less) or negative (as in eating unhealthy foods, eating too much or not enough, being sedentary, and stressing too often), create permanent readjustments within the fetus. In other words, a part of our genetic structure is cemented without our say.

Although the above scenario suggests that some people may have been dealt an unfair advantage in the gene pool— especially in their ability to accumulate body fat easily—it by no means indicates that any given situation is hopeless.

Instead, some people just have a little harder time than others. Your genes may be responsible for "loading the gun" when it comes to your present condition, but make no mistake about it, your diet, lifestyle, and environment are responsible for pulling the trigger.

The two-time Nobel Prize winner Dr. Linus Pauling said, "No crash diet or fad diet can solve the obesity problem, because these diets are so disagreeable and such a continuing nuisance that the obese person soon gives up. A successful treatment is one that will be adhered to year after year."

It's amazing to think that the majority of our population will subject themselves to these unhealthy Band-Aid approaches to losing excess body fat many times during their lifetime. Common sense would dictate that if the first few diets did not work, neither would the next few. And yet, as you read this, one-third of women and approximately one quarter of men can be found either starting or completing the latest fad diet. It's time to understand why we are failing so miserably at fat loss.

#1 Fitting Into Your Genes

Besides the fact that many individuals sit back and blame their "so-called" poor genes on their mom and pop (and their mom's and pop's mom and pop, and so on), there is a whole new area of science called *epigenetics*, which dictates that there is something above the genes that control who we become—it happens to be our mind.

Epigenetic researchers like former medical school professor Bruce Lipton, PhD, indicate that it is our perceptions— or too often our misperceptions of our environment (in other words, our belief system)—that actually control how our genes behave. And, all this time we were under the assumption that our genes control everything—WRONG! What this means is that you and you alone have the incredible ability to change your destiny;

all you have to do is change your belief system (more on this later).

> *"Forget about the consequences of failure. Failure is only a temporary change in direction to set you straight for your next success."*
>
> —*Denis Waitley*

#2 It's All About Balance

One of the main reasons so many people fail at losing body fat and maintaining a healthy metabolism is because they don't understand what got them to their present condition. It's important for those who are serious about living a long, lean life to first know how and why your body stores fat, and more importantly, how to mobilize that fat for energy. It is really about balance.

Any program that is overly restrictive or promises ridiculous results almost overnight is set for failure. What you need are effective, proven, and doable strategies that you can adhere to for life.

This is exactly what this book will give you, and as long as you are willing, able, and ready to apply these strategies, I can almost guarantee that you will finally be successful at Losing Fat 4 Life. But first, understand that no matter how many diets, exercise programs or magic formulas you have tried in your life, or how many times you have failed before, you *do* have the ability to change your life forever.

#3 Caution…Obesity Kills

It's never too late to reprogram your metabolism into a healthy, fat-burning machine. But, before I show you how to accomplish this in minimal time through my proven strategies, there is one very important question to ask yourself. Aside from cosmetic reasons, do you really know why it is so important to lose your excess body fat?

North Americans are getting progressively fatter every day. In the United States, well over 60 percent of the population is considered overly fat, and more than 50 percent of Canadians are too fat for their own good, with one-quarter of them being visually and clinically obese. Each year, the problem is worsening. In fact, even though we have indulged in copious amounts of delicious low-fat, no-fat foods that seem to line almost every shelf in our grocery stores today, our obesity rates have increased by a whopping 50 percent in the last 25 years. Since 1991, obesity has increased in every state of the United States, and every province of Canada, affecting both genders, all races, age groups, and educational levels. In other words, fat does not discriminate. And here's the kicker: more than 300,000 adults die in North America each year from conditions that are directly attributable to obesity (mortality figures one might expect from a major war).

"Ignorance is the curse of God; knowledge is the wing wherewith we fly to heaven."—William Shakespeare

#4 Not All Weight Is Created Equal

Before we go any further, let's clear up one very important issue. When it comes to your body, not all weight is created equal. The reason this statement is so important is that most individuals are concerned with how much they weigh, not how much body fat they carry. I have been telling people for years to throw away their bathroom scales. Why? Because they tell you absolutely nothing about your present condition, here's why:

Studies show that on most fad diets, the majority of people can expect to lose one pound of metabolically active tissue (lean body mass as in muscle) for every pound of body fat. So, at the end of their program they are basically no better off for their efforts. I call this the "smaller fat person" syndrome, because even though you may weigh less than when you started the diet, all you have done is become a smaller person—with the same amount of body fat!

#5 Muscle Is Your Metabolic Engine

This is one of the primary reasons that most chronic dieters almost always experience *rebound weight gain*. Rebound weight gain is when you gain back all the weight you previously lost on your diet and then a few extra pounds for insurance purposes! That is, insurance against another possible famine (to your brain, dieting and being without food means the same thing).

The point is, you can't afford to lose a single ounce of muscle. When you lose muscle, you lose your ability to burn calories (mostly fat) effectively and your metabolism slows down. This is because muscle is the key metabolic engine of the human body and the more muscle you have, the greater your ability to burn body fat. If you are going to continually lose muscle through dieting, (we also lose muscle through aging) you are continually going to degrade your metabolism (which is far from a wise thing to do). Hopefully, you now understand why it is so easy to regain lost pounds once you stop dieting.

#6 Don't Lose Weight—Lose Fat!

Imagine removing one of the sparkplugs from your car engine. Your car would be less efficient at burning fuel. Now imagine removing two then three and so on, I think you get the picture. The point is, when you continually lose muscle mass, it's like stripping your body of energy-producing spark plugs, which makes you less and less efficient at burning your own fat stores! The take-home message is simple: start differentiating where you want weight to come from. Instead of saying, "I want to lose weight," start saying, "I want to lose fat." Remember this: *a goal is defined by the detail of its description.*

You now realize that all weight is not created equal—so throw away that bathroom scale! A far more accurate way to judge your starting point, how you've progressed and when you've reached your final goal is to grab your tape measure.

Place the tape measure half way between the bottom of your rib cage and your hipbone.

For women an ideal waist measurement is between 28 and 33 inches. If your waist measurement is between 33 and 37 inches, you are in the overweight (over fat) category and if your measurement reads over 37 inches, you move into the obese category.

For men an ideal waist measurement is between 31 and 36 inches. If your waist measurement is between 36 and 40 inches, you are in the overweight (over fat) category and if your measurement reads over 40 inches, you move into the obese category.

> *"Our goals can only be reached through a vehicle of a plan, in which we must fervently believe, and upon which we must vigorously act.*

There is no other route to success."
—*Stephen A. Brennan*

#7 To Store or Not to Store

The human body is designed to do one of three things with the foods we consume: (1) burn some of the calories as immediate energy; (2) store what is not utilized immediately in its 30 billion fat cells; and (3) store some of the excess sugars from the diet as short-term energy, referred to as glycogen (long chains of sugar molecules), within the liver and skeletal muscles.

Here's where the story starts to unfold. The average human body only requires about one level teaspoon (5 grams) of blood sugar at any one time to run its millions of biochemical reactions. At the same time, our bodies only have the ability to store about half a day's worth of glycogen, which means we have a limited storage capacity for sugar.

#8 The Gatekeeper of Fat Storage

According to recent statistics from the Third National Health and Nutrition Examination Survey, the macronutrient that comprises the majority (50 percent) of our modern day diets comes from processed carbohydrates. By over consuming the wrong types of carbohydrates (and I am not talking about fruits and vegetables), you generate a rapid increase in blood sugar levels that in turn causes the pancreas to pump out loads of the hormone *insulin*. Insulin is essentially a storage hormone that not only lowers blood sugar, but also has a powerful message for your fat cells: STORE FAT!

Insulin accomplishes this task by stimulating a very powerful fat-storing enzyme called *lipoprotein lipase (LPL)*, which expands fat cells all the while making sure that fat doesn't get used as a fuel source. In fact, LPL is so good at its job that many obesity researchers refer to it as the *gatekeeper of fat storage*.

#9 Don't Let Your Diet Control You

Our bodies only have a limited storage capacity for carbohydrates. Therefore, any carbohydrates not used immediately by the body or stored as glycogen, are converted into triglycerides (the most prevalent form of fat in the body) and stored within the 30 billion fat cells throughout the body with the aid of LPL (and insulin of course). So, as you can see, food does not have to contain fat to become fat in your body.

Just as we can send our body messages for continual fat storage through the wrong dietary choices (i.e., excess high glycemic carbs), inactivity, and excess stress, we can also create the proper environment for continual fat loss by avoiding fat storing (processed) carbohydrates and consuming more fruits and vegetables, high quality proteins, and good fats.

The take-home message is clear: instead of allowing your diet to control you by placing your body in a fat storage environment, it's time you learned to control your diet and, thus, the fate of your metabolism.

> *"You wait for fate to bring about the changes in life which you should be bringing about by yourself."*
>
> —*Douglas Coupland*

CHAPTER 2

INSATIABLE CRAVINGS

The majority of diets would probably succeed—at least to some degree—if we were able to stay satisfied with them long enough to see the results. Many times, when people make a commitment to lose the excess body fat (the old "this time I'm serious" syndrome), it is usually those insatiable cravings for the sweet, starchy, fatty foods that get the best of them. So why do we seem to always have the same cravings for the very foods that make us fat and keep us there? Because many of us experience unbalanced or low brain chemicals such as *serotonin* (more on this a little later), we have low or wild fluctuations in blood sugar levels or we follow the most extreme method to weight loss (i.e., crazy dieting)—all of which lead to undesirable constant cravings.

#10 Oh No, Not another Famine!

Most of us forget that it takes months and years to gain unwanted pounds, yet we want the extra weight gone yesterday! We reduce our calories to the point of actually slowing our metabolism, we get rid of all the fat (forgetting that the brain is 60 percent fat) and raise our fat-converting carbohydrates through the roof or we get rid of the carbs altogether. When we take the "all or nothing approach" to dieting, we offset the intricate biochemical balance of the body and invariably create cravings that cannot be ignored.

As it pertains to how fast your present metabolism is, the size of your appetite may mean a lot more than the size of your meals! In other words, your body's ability to store extra fat may be directly linked to the degree to which you desire and crave foods rather than solely the degree to which you consume them. Why? Insatiable cravings send false starvation signals to your body, switching it into an extreme fat-storing mode. In this state, your body slows its metabolic rate and stops "burning" excess calories, opting to stockpile them for a perceived famine.

#11 Hormonal Mayhem

The majority of our cravings are due to extreme fluctuations in our blood sugar levels. The higher the glycemic (simple sugars) carbohydrates we consume (even when they are void of fat) like, grains, pastas, and even fruit juices, the more dramatic is the rise in our storage hormone insulin. High blood sugar levels and high insulin levels create a hypoglycemic (low blood sugar) response due to the higher half-life of insulin, which tends to remain active even after blood sugar levels are lowered.

This initiates a craving response in the brain for sweet, carbohydrate-rich foods that are able to raise blood sugar levels once again. This rise and fall of insulin and blood sugar also creates an enhanced environment conducive to continual fat storage. This is created by preventing the metabolism of fats for energy, and instead sets into play the usage of sugars and proteins as the main fuel sources.

#12 The Macronutrient Balance

Without a steady supply of other macronutrients such as high quality protein, fiber, and essential fatty acids (omega-3 and omega-6), our bodies cannot deal with the onslaught of excess sugars as they are broken down into glucose (a simple sugar).

Protein and essential fatty acids are responsible for boosting your metabolism by stimulating the release of the hormone glucagon, which helps to balance blood sugar and stimulate the necessary enzymes for fat burning. Fibers help to regulate insulin levels by slowing the release of sugars into your system, all the while enhancing your cells' ability to accept sugars from the bloodstream (insulin sensitivity).

#13 Nutrient Deficiencies

There is some evidence that certain cravings may reflect a primitive mechanism within the body, which uses appetite to guide a person to foods containing the missing or needed elements. It is suggested that bizarre cravings for food combinations (i.e., ice cream and pickles) may actually have a rational biological explanation once all the elements are considered. As the late Dr. Lendon Smith pointed out in his bestselling book, <u>Feed Your Body Right</u>, pregnancy cravings for foods like ice cream may represent a need for extra calcium, while pickles would represent the need for acid to absorb the calcium.

We also know that chocolate is the most frequently craved of all foods, especially during a woman's menstrual cycle. This may be in part due to a magnesium deficiency, as treatment with magnesium has been shown to reduce chocolate cravings. Another important nutrient is the trace mineral chromium, which is essential in normal carbohydrate and lipid metabolism. Chromium deficiency can lead to elevated insulin levels, which then creates a low blood sugar environment, creating the need for more sugar. The interesting thing is that most of our soils are depleted of this essential element causing a possible deficiency in the majority of the population. Many excessive sugar eaters (i.e., processed food) lose a tremendous amount of chromium through their urine as a by-product of metabolizing the sugar.

#14 More Deficiencies

Excess sugars in the body also act like a vacuum for B Vitamins. Without the B vitamins, your body cannot produce efficient energy or manufacture the necessary neurochemicals for proper brain functions (one of the reasons B vitamins are so important in alleviating some depressive states).

For instance, a deficiency of vitamin B12, which according to one of the longest running studies (the Framingham study) is believed to affect almost half of the US population, can disrupt our ability to produce energy. Any disruption in our energy cycle will greatly disturb our ability to burn fat, which is yet another way in which the wrong carbohydrates can cause fat to accumulate.

#15 Brain Chemical Imbalances

Our bodies have a remarkable way of self-medicating themselves. When we are feeling down, depressed, or stressed out, we instantly reach for the sweetest foods we can find. One of the reasons for this is dietary sugars stimulate insulin release, and by elevating insulin, we are able to raise certain levels of brain chemicals called neurotransmitters (chemicals that relay messages from one neuron to the next) that culminate in a sigh of relief.

Unfortunately, this escapade quickly dissipates and the brain calls out for more sugary medication (i.e., sweets or starches). By stimulating insulin (through carbohydrate intake), the brain is able to temporarily raise levels of the neurotransmitter serotonin, which balances our moods by creating feelings of calmness and satiety to the rest of the body. Out of 40 known neurotransmitters, serotonin is the most important in terms of appetite, cravings, and sleep.

#16 Serotonin Deficiency Syndrome

Balanced serotonin levels are important in any fat loss program because they provide a calming and appetite suppressing action, which allows you to feel satisfied without needing to cheat. When serotonin levels rise, we feel instant gratification in the reward centers of the brain. Serotonin levels decline throughout the day and are replenished during the sleep phase.

Many people who have sleep difficulties also have serotonin deficiencies (also referred to as the serotonin deficiency syndrome). This would also account for why people, who consistently stay up late, tend to binge-eat the most.

#17 Stress and Appetite

Serotonin levels are also quickly depleted during times of stress. And with the stressful lives we subject ourselves to day in and day out, it is not hard to imagine our serotonin tanks are running on half-empty at most times. As mentioned earlier, serotonin levels are increased in response to high carbohydrate foods, especially those that break down into sugars rapidly, but why? Blood sugar raises the hormone insulin and insulin creates an easy access to the main building block of serotonin, tryptophan.

When you raise insulin in response to incoming sugars (carbohydrates), the insulin lowers the blood sugar along with all the amino acids in the blood except one, tryptophan. This elimination of the competition allows tryptophan to pass through the blood–brain barrier and induce a feeling of calmness and satiety, but only for a short while. Before you know it, your brain is once again screaming for its carbohydrate fix.

#18 All or Nothing Never Works

Thankfully, by consuming a proper balance of protein, fibers, and essential fatty acids (along with low-glycemic carbohydrates) at regular intervals throughout the day (eating approximately every 2.5–3 hours), you can stabilize blood sugar levels and create a proper balance between insulin and glucagon.

This is why the all or nothing scenario never works for long. It always offsets the homeostasis (balance) of the body and cravings ensue. For extra-craving control, the eating principles outlined in this book provide a blend of the right nutrients designed to help control insulin and blood sugar levels, balance neurotransmitters, and eliminate insatiable cravings that put the brakes on fat loss. When you eliminate these nasty cravings—you give your body the advantage it needs to continually place your metabolism in your control.

> *"Cravings and urges only last a few minutes. If you can distract those, chances are you will get past it."—Susan Gibbons*

Chapter 3

REVVING THE ENGINE

In Chapters 1 and 2, you learned about
the importance of your muscle tissue in
maintaining your metabolic advantage. I
explained that losing muscle mass is like
removing the spark plugs from your
engine. At the end of the day, your
body's metabolism has a difficult time
using fat as its premiere energy source,
period! If your muscle cells are akin to
the spark plugs that burn your car's fuel,
then your thyroid gland—and its
hormones—are akin to the timing
mechanism that determines how

efficiently that fuel gets burned. As you are about to find out, the health of your thyroid gland and how effective your body is at producing a special brain chemical can often be the missing piece of your fat loss puzzle.

#19 The Little Gland that Could

Your thyroid gland, which is located in the front of the neck attached to the lower part of the voice box (or larynx), is like the master controller of your metabolism. With the aid of its specialized hormones, *thyroxin* (T4) and *triiodothyronine* (T3), this gland is responsible for controlling your overall metabolism. Thyroid hormones control numerous metabolic functions, including body temperature, the release of energy from cells and your body's ability to repair itself effectively.

Ninety-three percent of the hormones produced by the thyroid are in the form of the relatively inactive T4 hormone. In order to lose fat for life, these hormones must be converted into the much more metabolically active T3 hormone. Aside from the fact that many dieters lose too much muscle, one of the reasons most diets fail, especially the excessively low calorie ones, is due to a drop in this hormone conversion, which ultimately leads to a slowdown in overall metabolism (and rebound weight gain).

#20 Love Your Liver

Unfortunately, many people, especially women, experience a glitch in the machine when it comes to their ability to produce sufficient quantities of thyroid hormones. It is the thyroid hormones' ability to readily convert into the metabolically active T3 hormone that fires up your metabolism.

The great majority of metabolically active T3 is produced outside of the thyroid gland, within the liver (and to a lesser extent the kidneys). This can pose a problem in today's day and age due to the never-ending job the liver has when it comes to keeping our systems clean (the liver is your body's major detoxification organ). For instance, numerous toxins, excess hormones, and/or high fat/high sugar meals can greatly burden the liver's activities, thereby reducing its ability to produce sufficient quantities of T3. Aside from this, many people experience a dysfunctional thyroid gland with age, leading to lower and lower levels of T3. Research also indicates that many people experience a decline in the conversion of T4 to active T3 with advancing age.

#21 Hypothyroidism

The late thyroid expert, Dr. Broda Barnes, author of Hypothyroidism: The Unsuspected Illness (Harper Collins), estimated that over one-third of the adult North American population suffered from a subclinical thyroid deficiency or hypothyroidism that robbed them of their full metabolic potential. To support this theory, research from the Oregon Health Sciences University in Portland showed that elderly people, who were found to have normal thyroid activity in standard tests, were later found to have serious thyroid deficiencies after undergoing advanced testing.

Indications that your thyroid production might be deficient include uncontrolled weight gain, difficulty losing weight, constant fatigue, depression, cold intolerance, dry skin, brittle fingernails and hair, constipation, heart disease, high cholesterol, and poor memory.

Basal Metabolic Test

If you suspect that you may have a low thyroid status (hypothyroidism) and your lab tests have been negative, try this at-home test to assess your thyroid function:

Have a thermometer beside your bed and take your temperature first thing in the morning before you get up, while you are lying in bed and are as relaxed as possible. (Normal resting temperature in the morning is between **97.8** and **98.2** degrees Fahrenheit.) Record the results. Take your temperature later in the day as well. (Normal active body temperature is **98.6** degrees Fahrenheit.) Also, record the results. Because hormone fluctuations will alter body temperature, women should start recording body temperature on the first day of menstruation.

Take your temperature anywhere from three to five days. Below average body temperature suggests functional low thyroid status, while higher than average temperature suggests a functional high thyroid status (hyperthyroidism).

#22 The Four Corners of Optimal Thyroid Health

Although the thyroid gland requires numerous nutrients to continually operate at peak efficiency, I have chosen four nutrients that have been scientifically validated to enhance the overall effectiveness of the thyroid gland and its hormones (look for formulas that contain synergistic combinations of these thyroid-supportive nutrients):

1) *L-tyrosine*: An amino acid that is a direct precursor to your thyroid hormones. Deficiencies of tyrosine are known to cause hypothyroidism.

2) *Selenium*: This mineral is essential to the conversion of T4 to T3 (the enzyme responsible for T3 production is a selenium-containing enzyme). Unfortunately, selenium is highly deficient in our soils throughout North America.

3) *Iodine*: Iodine is needed by the body to form thyroid hormones. Look for naturally derived and preferably organic forms of iodine (sea vegetables are a great source).

4) *Guggulsterones*: Guggulsterones are derived from the sticky gum resin of the Asian mukul myrrh tree. Guggulsterones have been documented traditionally to treat disorders of fat metabolism, including obesity. These incredible phytonutrients support thyroid health by increasing the conversion of T4 to T3.

#23 Signaling Fat Loss with Norepinephrine

Your fat cells store fat in bundles of three fatty acids called *triglycerides*. In order to become fuel for the body, these triglycerides must first be broken down into simple fatty acids and then transported to the engines of your muscle cells (called *mitochondria*), where they are burned or oxidized as energy.

Your body uses chemical messengers referred to as neurotransmitters—such as *epinephrine* and *norepinephrine*—to tell your body to begin breaking down the fat. Unfortunately, your body doesn't like a lot of fat to be wasted (especially if you have a dysfunctional metabolism), so it often creates an enzyme to break down these chemical messengers, which means putting the brakes on fat burning.

#24 Caffeine—Good or Bad?

Chemical messengers like norepinephrine often decline as we age, gain weight, or go on a diet. In fact, research presented in the *American Journal of Clinical Nutrition* indicated that norepinephrine levels often drop by close to 50 percent when you lose just 10 percent of your bodyweight. A reduction in norepinephrine is one of the primary reasons fat loss seems to stop the longer you stay on most diets.

Needless to say, norepinephrine is a friend to your metabolism—that is as long as it is not over-stimulated (which causes an unwanted rise in stress hormones). One of the ways people unknowingly stimulate this brain chemical is by consuming caffeine-laced beverages like coffee (the number one consumed beverage in North America). The problem is that we often over consume these beverages and any positive effects our metabolism may experience from the caffeine is quickly overridden by the excess stress hormones that hang around afterwards, which in the end, degrade our metabolism.

> **Metabolic Stimulants**
>
> One of the ways in which caffeine helps to stimulate metabolism, is by inhibiting the enzyme responsible for breaking norepinephrine down. This is one of the primary reasons metabolic stimulants or "fat burners" contain caffeine—to stimulate norepinephrine levels in order to send fat releasing signals to your fat cells. Research from the Department of Human Nutrition in Copenhagen, Denmark, suggests that when norepinephrine levels are increased, there is a substantial increase in the number of fat calories used each day.

#25 Burn Fat With Chocolate—Say What!!!

Some well-designed natural metabolic formulas include a different kind of caffeine that has been documented to be more effective at helping to raise norepinephrine levels (and are safer) than regular caffeine (from coffee). Ever wonder what makes you feel so good when you eat chocolate (women, I'm talking especially to you)? Chocolate contains a phytonutrient called *theobromine* that is ultimately responsible for that "feel good" sensation.

Theobromine, from the Brazilian cocoa bean contains *methylxanthine*—a chemical relative of caffeine. However, because of its unique chemical structure (it contains three methyl groups instead of two found in regular caffeine), it is slower reacting than caffeine—ultimately working to raise norepinephrine levels over a longer period of time. And the more norepinephrine circulating in your system, the more fat your body gets to release—and ultimately burn for energy. Imagine the benefits of chocolate, without the added sugar and fat!

#26 Feeling Good Naturally—The Methylation Connection

What good would a life-changing fat loss program be if it didn't help you feel better in the process. Let's face it, your moods affect your habits and your habits eventually become your destiny. In this case, your destiny is designed around your new fat-burning metabolism. In order to feel our best, we sometimes need a little help from a biochemical process that goes on every day inside our cells even though we are probably not aware of it.

Methylation—the transfer of methyl groups (CH3) within our bodies—is a biochemical process imperative to good health, especially where metabolism and mental function is concerned. Substances that aid in methylation are called methyl donors, which are necessary for maintaining healthy brain cell metabolism and helping manufacture adequate neurotransmitters (yes, even norepinephrine). According to Craig Cooney, PhD, the author of the book Methyl Magic, we cannot maintain sufficient methylation as we age without supplementation because today's diet does not supply a sufficient amount of methyl groups.

#27 It's Time to Get Methylated?

Because modern research indicates that many of us (perhaps everyone) may indeed be deficient in specific nutrients that support optimal methylation, it stands to reason that supplementing one's diet with these nutrients (whether in a high-quality multivitamin or on their own) may help support healthy metabolism.

The chief methyl donors (and don't even try to pronounce the first two) are: *S-adenosylmethionine* (SAMe), *trimethylglycine* (TMG), *choline*, *folic acid*, *vitamin B6*, and *vitamin B12*. Studies have shown that methyl donors like SAMe, TMG, and folic acid act as powerful natural antidepressants.

In fact, researchers from Finland have concluded that men who have the lowest dietary folate (folic acid) intake have a 67 percent greater risk of suffering from depression than those with the highest intake. Further research shows that folic acid supplementation (as little as 500 mcg) can greatly improve one's response to conventional antidepressants like *fluoxetine* (Prozac®). This makes a lot of sense since studies show that almost 50 percent of those suffering from depression also exhibit high levels of *homocysteine*—a by-product of insufficient methylation.

CHAPTER 4

STRESS AND YOUR METABOLISM

Many of the top medical researchers around the world agree that stress may be the number one reason why so many people are sick nowadays. The body produces many powerful hormones during stress response—the main ones being *adrenaline* and *cortisol* (both produced from your adrenal glands). It is adrenaline that causes your heart rate and muscular strength to increase and heighten your senses. Adrenaline also happens to be one of the largest contributors to premature aging, as it is one of the strongest oxidizing agents known. But, did you know that excess stress can often lead to a dysfunctional metabolism that makes it next to impossible to lose body fat?

#28 Anabolic/Catabolic—The Two Sides of Metabolism

Hormones regulate many metabolic events in the body. Some of our hormones are *anabolic*, as they help to build body tissues—*testosterone* and *growth hormone* comes to mind—while other hormones are *catabolic*, as they stimulate the breakdown of body tissues (i.e., muscle). When we constantly expose ourselves to stress in our day-to-day lives, or rely on too many metabolic stimulants like coffee to get us through each day, we end up creating a highly catabolic state that eventually reduces our metabolic ability (think, "I can't lose the fat no matter what I try!").

The most well known catabolic hormone is cortisol. Cortisol levels should be their highest in the morning and lowest in the evening (who can fall asleep when they are stressed out?). Due to present day lifestyles, cortisol levels can remain elevated over extended periods of time. Not a wise thing where your metabolism is concerned as muscle is quickly destroyed in a high cortisol state.

#29 Stress Eats Protein

When the body recognizes a new stress, whether actual or perceived, it releases large amounts of adrenaline and cortisol. These two hormones are responsible for the famous "fight-or-flight" response we inherited from our ancestors. By up-regulating our stress hormones in times of need, we can quickly break down sugars, dietary fats, and dietary proteins into their simplest components in order to supply enough energy to our cellular engines—so we can theoretically fight or flee!

In order to access some of that energy, when instructed by cortisol, your body uses protein. If there isn't a supply of dietary protein (amino acids) in the system, cortisol will have no other choice but to take it from your own body and your valuable muscle tissue will be the first to go. This spells long-term damage to your metabolism and is one of the primary reasons you gain back all the weight you've lost—and then some—after most diets. Cortisol eats away at the muscle that is used to burn fat. Here's an easy equation to remember: excess stress equals excess cortisol, which often equals fat gain. (And we thought we gained weight during times of high stress because we chow down on all that comfort food.)

#30 Diets Create Stress

The fact is that any loss of muscle is a victory for the fat side. Fat wins every time you lose even an ounce of muscle. To spare muscle, you've got to reduce the level of cortisol and/or raise your level of anabolic hormones. I've already mentioned that cortisol is increased during a reduced-calorie diet or fasting—which is one more reason most diets don't work! The more unreasonably you restrict yourself on a diet, the more stress is felt by the body and the more cortisol is produced.

Almost every one of your body's 100 trillion-plus cells can burn either fat or glucose as fuel, but the brain—under non-fasting conditions—relies heavily on available glucose for energy. Your brain uses almost one-half of your body's total blood sugar (approximately 100 grams) per day. Unlike the other organs of the body, which require insulin to pump glucose into their interiors, your brain is able to absorb glucose independent of insulin, which gives it first priority over the other cells of the body. That is, unless insulin levels are kept chronically high through consumption of insulin-spiking carbs all day long and staying up late in the evening.

#31 Stress and Insulin Resistance

The hormone glucagon—stimulated by protein—is responsible for raising low blood sugar levels, thus allowing sugar to remain accessible to the brain. If glucagon can't do its job properly because high levels of circulating insulin are blocking its actions, then the brain must look at alternate routes of accessibility. Your brain must take whatever steps it needs to ensure its primary fuel supply; even if it means the other cells of the body are deprived of sugar. This is where cortisol enters the picture.

Cortisol—in addition to cannibalizing existing body structures to make glucose—decreases the amount of glucose used by other cells, ultimately causing insulin resistance, which means more fat and the eventuality of diabetes.

#32 Stress lowers Metabolic Hormones

Cortisol is produced along the same biochemical pathway as other hormones, and during stressful times, excess cortisol is manufactured at the expense of other healthful hormones like *dihydroepiandrosterone* (DHEA) and *testosterone*. Both DHEA and testostcrone are needed to maintain and grow muscle tissue and if you haven't got the message by now, without muscle, fat cannot be burned.

DHEA is also needed to maintain a healthy metabolism. In fact, research at the University of Wisconsin, Madison, has shown that derivatives of DHEA help start thermogenesis (the burning of body fat), and may help decrease the incidence of obesity. Since one of the most important roles DHEA has is in balancing the effects of cortisol, perhaps this is one of the keys to its metabolism-enhancing effects

#33 Belly Fat Loves Stress

The longer you maintain a stress response, the more body fat you accumulate—especially in the abdominal cavity. One of the main reasons for this is because abdominal fat is loaded with cortisol receptors. In fact, abdominal fat has on average, four times the amount of cortisol receptors than any other fat containing area within the body.

Abdominal fat poses a double whammy to your metabolism. Not only does it have more of an affinity for cortisol, but research presented in the journal *Diabetes* indicates that abdominal fat can also contribute substantially to the regeneration of cortisol—ouch!

#34 Stress and Serotonin

Researchers have discovered that one of the main reasons we crave carbohydrates is to compensate for a reduction in serotonin levels, which help make us feel better (those "comfort foods" get us every time). Carbohydrates elevate brain serotonin by stimulating insulin levels, which ultimately drive the amino acid tryptophan—the main building block of serotonin—into the brain. This is also believed to be one of the primary reasons we crave carbohydrates when we are feeling down or are experiencing excess stress (depression and stress can greatly deplete tryptophan levels), in order to compensate for lower than normal serotonin levels at these times.

Brain serotonin levels are quickly depleted when we are under excess stress. This is due to an increase in various enzymes that gobble up an enormous amount of tryptophan (the building block of serotonin) in order to use it to make other substances the body believes are more important during stressful times. As you can see, stress and serotonin (and also sleep) are intricately linked.

#35 Change Your Perceptions

Along with cortisol's effect on degrading your metabolic engines—muscle—cortisol has also been shown to affect the memory-producing center of the brain by destroying *hippocampal* neurons. As mentioned, cortisol levels are elevated during many life stresses (i.e., illness, in-laws visits, work-induced panic attacks, being caught in a traffic jam, losing a job, losing a loved one, or having too many bills to deal with). You're pumping out stress hormones daily, often with no letup or release. And often, you're stressed over anticipated events rather than actual ones.

Anyway you look at it, stress is stress, whether it's real or imaginary. Mark Twain said it best: "*I have been through some terrible things in my life, some of which actually happened.*" In order to win the war on fat and create an optimum, healthy environment, you have to change your perception of reality, and learn to face many of the events in your life with some degree of calm.

#36 Don't Overreact

Starting today make sure to have more fun in life and not perceive it as overly stressful. Remember that your body responds the same to mental and emotional stress as it does to physical stress. So, it doesn't matter whether the threat is actual or perceived. Please take time for yourself to reflect your state of mind.

Whenever you are faced with a possible stressful trigger (traffic jam, an annoying person, another bill, etc.) take a second to reflect on the situation and instantly break the cycle by following these three simple steps: (1) instantly look up, (2) take a deep breath right from your belly, and (3) smile, and if you can let out a big laugh. Trust me, these are the tools many an expert dealing in stress-psychology will share with you for a lot more than you paid for this book.

CHAPTER 5

SLEEP AND YOUR METABOLISM

What would you say if I was to tell you that healthy fat-burning metabolism was dependent on a good night's sleep? That's right, your body's ability to burn fat each day is to a large extent controlled by how effectively you are able to sleep and restore your metabolic activity for the next day. According to the latest research from the National Institutes of Health, Cornell University, and the Sansum Medical Research Institute in Santa Barbara, California (where insulin was first synthesized), in order to lose excess body fat, slow biological aging and perform at peak energy efficiency, one must get enough quality sleep, period!

#37 Loss of Sleep Makes You Fat

No matter how you look at it, sleep deprivation makes you fat. Dozens of research studies dating back from decades ago confirm the sleep–weight connection. Warwick Medical School scientists found that severe sleep deprivation nearly *doubles* your risk of being obese. However, it doesn't take all-nighters for this phenomenon to set in and take hold. Simply sleeping less than seven hours dramatically boosts your chances of being fat.

Any doubts about sleep's influence on fat accumulation were put to rest when a group of scientists gathered data from 1.1 million research subjects. The researchers concluded that anything less than eight hours contributes substantially to making you overweight, and less than six makes you obese. In the case of sleep and fatness, there's plenty of substantiated research that points to less sleep equals more fat.

#38 Sleep is Not a Passive State

How can sleep, a state where you're doing practically nothing, have such a profound impact on your ability to lose the pounds? It turns out that the common belief that sleep is a passive state is dead wrong! Sleep is actually a highly active and complex state and many of the control systems that impact sleep still remain a mystery.

While the physiology of sleep has become somewhat unraveled (largely due to the emerging area of "sleep science"), one of the most surprising discoveries is just how much sleep influences how healthy your metabolism is. Many scientists are under the assumption that sleep deprivation sends evolutionary fat-storing signals to the body. In hunter-gatherer times, food was more plentiful in the summer months when plants were at their peak ripeness and animals were not hibernating. Your body may associate a shortened sleep time as a signal to store fat and eat everything in sight for the long winter months ahead. In other words, take advantage of the buffet while you can.

#39 Hormonal Rhythms

Twenty-four hour hormonal regulation lies within our biological clock, which is located in an area of the brain called the hypothalamus. This biological clock—the *suprachiasmatic nuclei* (don't even try to pronounce this one)—orchestrates the rise and fall in all of our hormones throughout the day and night. When we allow ourselves to become out of sync with nature's clock by staying up late into the evening or missing valuable sleep, our hormonal rhythms begin to run amuck and in the process our metabolism begins to decline.

In the evening, our sex hormones should be at an all day low, along with our stress hormones. The "rose" light of the setting sun should automatically trigger the release of your sleep hormone (and the most powerful antioxidant known to man) *melatonin*. Melatonin lowers your body temperature (which is one of the reasons you need a blanket to sleep, even in the summer), which in turn lowers your stress hormones (i.e., cortisol) and readies your body for a deep restorative night of sleep. Or at least this is what nature intended for us.

#40 Sleep Loss and Appetite

Studies show that even a single night of subpar sleep makes you hungrier the next day. As the "sleep debt" grows, so does your craving for sugary foods. Research at the University of Chicago forced a group of men to limit their sleep in the laboratory to just four hours. The next day, their appetite and hunger levels shot up 25 percent. The amazing thing was that these sleep-deprived volunteers had insatiable cravings for sweet and salty foods and were not even remotely interested in fruits and veggies. After crunching some numbers, one of the researchers estimated that if left alone to eat whatever they wanted, they'd consume an extra 500 calories per day.

Why does pulling an all-nighter do such a number on our appetite? First off, when you're tired, you tend to reach for comfort foods like chocolate, ice cream, or chips. These comfort foods stimulate a great deal of insulin, which helps tryptophan get into the brain where it can make serotonin and melatonin—your sleep hormone.

#41 Becoming Insulin Resistant

A dysfunction with our insulin system, or insulin resistance, is a well-known cause of obesity. In fact, well over 90 percent of Type 2 diabetics are obese. One of the most alarming effects of sleep deprivation is its impact on insulin resistance. Scientists have understood that sleep deprivation, obesity, and diabetes are usually found in tandem. Obesity is the prime risk factor for a sleep-impairing condition called *obstructive sleep apnea*, which *also* throws off insulin and exacerbates the problem.

People who have diabetes also tend to suffer from obstructive sleep apnea (OSA) and research now shows that all it takes is a few nights of sleep deprivation to create a diabetic state. In one study, researchers curbed the sleep time of young men of healthy weight to six hours a night. After about a week, they became so insulin resistant that if you were to look at their lab results, you'd think they were diabetic. Less sleep = more insulin = more fat.

#42 Don't Take Drugs to Sleep

North Americans handover more than $4.5 billion every year for drugs that *supposedly* help them sleep. Popularity aside, there remains a question of whether these things work as they claim. Despite their ridiculous price tag, very few studies have found that they lengthen the duration of deep sleep. In fact, The National Institute of Health recently found that a battery of "cutting edge" sleeping pills like *Ambien*, *Lunesta*, and *Sonata* only boost sleep time by about 10 minutes.

What about the side effects? Regular users have reported amnesia and addiction as a common problem, with one class of sleeping pills called *benzodiazepines* being especially habit-forming. Unfortunately, all sleeping pills hit your brain's addiction centers on two fronts: physiological and psychological. Sleeping pills are drugs, so there's a certain level of chemical dependency that inevitably occurs over time. The verdict: don't take them!

#43 The Natural Way to Help You Sleep

Unlike sleeping pills, which are synthetic sedatives, there are natural alternatives that are non-addicting and actually work. The following are some of my favorites:

Melatonin: Research from *The Lancet* found that "Melatonin deficiency may have an important role in the high frequency of insomnia..." and that popping melatonin before bedtime significantly improved sleep quality.

Griffonia: This is a shrub extract that has high levels of a natural form of *5-Hydroxytryptophan* (5HTP), the activated form of tryptophan that's especially important for serotonin and melatonin.

Theanine: This is found in high concentrations in tea, and has the unique ability of "smoothing" out erratic brainwaves, as confirmed by EEG.

Ziziphus: Also known as *Jujube*, this compound contains special chemicals called *sapponins*, that bring on relaxation.

Hops extract: It has been compared in studies with a prescription strength benzodiazepine drug and found to work just as well and with zero reports of side effects.

Valerian: This herb that was spoken about by Hippocrates, the father of modern medicine, has been found to shorten the time it takes to get to sleep and seems to make sleep more refreshing overall.

#44 Turn the Lights Out

In today's day and age, we often interfere with our melatonin production—often unknowingly—by stressing out throughout the day (remember those tryptophan-gobbling enzymes?), consuming the wrong foods (primarily protein deficient convenience foods), staying up too late or subjecting ourselves to violent television shows, or too much light before bed. All of these things have a pronounced effect on your body and your brain's ability to manufacture adequate levels of melatonin in order to help you replenish and repair your cells metabolic activity.

For optimum sleep to occur, the darker the environment, the better. This means sleeping without any lights on whatsoever (including night lights, clock radio lights, TV lights, etc.). Sleep is the greatest asset you have to burn excess body fat. It is the time when we switch from a catabolic breakdown state, to that of an anabolic rebuilding one. *Human growth hormone* (HGH)—a very powerful weapon in the war against body fat—controls much of this anabolic state. The amazing reality is that approximately 75 percent of HGH is produced while we are in our deepest phase of sleep—the delta phase.

#45 Recommended Tips for Creating an Optimal Sleep Environment

- Limit your bedroom use to sleep and sex. This means no watching television or anything else that will stimulate your brain and make sleep more difficult.

- Make sure your bed is as comfortable as possible and find the perfect sleeping temperature.
- Don't be frugal when it comes to purchasing your perfect bed; after all, it's probably the most important investment you'll ever make.
- Be as regular as possible with your sleep times, even on the weekends. Anything more than an hour off of your regular sleep schedule can throw your biological clock into a tail spin.
- Dim the lights in the evening.
- Take a warm shower if you are having trouble sleeping. This not only relaxes your muscles, but also lowers your body temperature once out of the shower, creating an optimal environment for sleep.
- Avoid caffeine, nicotine, and alcohol in the late afternoon and evening.
- Only nap—and for no longer than a half hour—if you are unable to get enough continuous sleep at night.

- Don't exercise too late in the evening. Late bouts of exercise raise your body's temperature and will signal your body to stay awake.
- Leave at least three hours between exercise and bed.
- Expose yourself to bright lights in the morning. Sunlight resets your biological clock.
- Consume proven natural non-habit-forming sleep formulas—such as Ultimate Sleep.

Chapter 6

WATER YOU MADE OF?

Any way you look at it, you are mostly water! Your brain and muscles are three-quarters water. Your blood and lungs are more than 80 percent water. Even your bones are one-quarter water. Next to oxygen, water is unquestionably the most important nutrient for sustaining life. The problem is that too many of us take it for granted and don't drink enough water. The question is, if you take water for granted, aren't you in essence taking yourself for granted?

Well, you might say, "I drink plenty of liquids: juice, coffee, tea, sodas." Nothing can take the place of water. A great many of us may indeed be dehydrated and not even know it! Aging is a process of drying out, so is obesity. Many health researchers and medical experts now believe that water—not just fluid—is essential to our health and well-being, and is key to slowing down the aging process and helping us lose excess body fat!

#46 Muscle is Mostly Water

The great majority of North Americans will lose anywhere from one-third to one-half of their lean body mass over their lifetimes—especially if they are sedentary (resistance exercise maintains muscle). According to Dr. Robert Mazzeo, professor of exercise physiology at the University of Colorado, the majority of major health risks for the frail elderly are immobility, falls, and fractures, which are all related to muscle weakness. Studies prove that maintaining and enhancing muscle mass is associated with increased energy, lower body fat levels, better moods, stronger connective tissue, better immunity—and the list goes on. As you are now aware, your muscles are 75 percent water.

Speaking of experiencing more energy and less body fat, everyone realizes how important regular exercise is. Intensive exercise can cause a person to lose five to eight pounds of fluid through perspiration, evaporation, and exhalation. Studies show that for every pound of fluid lost, there is a significant drop in the efficiency with which the body produces energy. Everybody wants energy! But, how many of us actually understand how energy is made in the body?

#47 Energy 101

Most energy is produced in tiny little power plants within our cells called *mitochondria* (my-toe-con-dria). The more active a cell is, the more mitochondria it contains. Some of our cells (such as heart, muscle, and brain cells) contain thousands of these tiny power plants. Our cells are completely dependent upon mitochondria to sustain life by generating energy.

The mitochondria are also where the majority of your fat is burned as energy. They produce power through a process called the Krebs cycle. This cycle is responsible for converting nutrients from the food we eat—the protein, carbs, and fats—into a universal chemical energy substance called ATP (*adenosine triphosphate*). ATP is like an electrical source: nothing in our body runs without it. In fact, we use so much ATP on a daily basis that the total amount required just to get most of us through the day would weigh in at an estimated 150 to 200 pounds.

#48 Creating Hydroelectricity

The process by which ATP is converted from our foods into the energy we feel is extremely complicated. So complicated that we still don't fully understand (or can we recreate) how the body manufactures energy using a process called electron transfer.

So what does all this biochemistry babble have to do with water, you ask? The fact remains that water is imperative in the creation of ATP. In fact, ATP has to be broken down by water in order to generate energy—in a process called hydrolysis (meaning "water broken"). As I have mentioned before, ATP is like an electrical charge, and water is responsible for providing the primary hydroelectric energy that is stored in ATP when the cell is inactive. As your cells become active, water hydrolyzes ATP, and energy is released again so that you can do everything it is you do during a 24-hour period–yes, even sleep! As you can imagine, a low water environment means inadequate energy production and less efficient metabolism.

#49 Hungry for Water

Water may also be an important way to control hunger pangs. Many researchers believe that we have lost our biological ability to discern thirst from hunger, a condition exacerbated by age and obesity. It is theorized that somewhere in our evolutionary past, the signals for the two (hunger and thirst) may have crossed wires. In other words, when you feel hungry, you may actually be thirsty. Thus, by keeping yourself properly hydrated, you can avoid false cravings for food.

Imagine if during the times when you feel that insatiable urge to eat, you are actually thirsty. This is one of the reasons I recommend consuming a full glass of water (8 oz.) approximately 15 minutes prior to eating. If your body was indeed low on water, it will help curb your appetite.

#50 Detoxifying with Water

If you're still not convinced as to why nothing can take the place of water, read on. Water helps the body eliminate toxins, the waste products that accumulate in our systems. If you have ever tried to lose excess body fat, are you aware of what also gets lost in your tissues?

When your 30 billion fat cells release their fat as energy, they also evict tremendous amounts of fat-soluble toxins that are lodged in that fat. And guess what? Your system needs water to help detoxify these toxins before they can take up residence once more in your fat cells and cause further damage to your body—especially your hormonal system. One study published in the *Journal of Lipid Research* showed that unwanted weight gain (excess body fat) may be strongly linked to hormone-disrupting contaminants that can accumulate in fat cells.

#51 Is Tap Water Good Enough?

Many of those hormone-disrupting contaminants I touched on in the last section are actually found in plastic bottles, which is one of the reasons (that and the environmental impact) I highly advise against buying your water in them. One of these hormonal-disrupters is BPH (*bisphenol-A*), which has been shown to cause fat cells to both expand and increase in numbers. But, what about tap water?

Have you ever left a few drops of tap water in a glass on your counter only to come back to a dried residue of sediment? Do you actually believe that the sediment should be in your body—it shouldn't! More than 60,000 different chemicals are known to contaminate our water supplies, and studies show that we each may drink more than 450 pounds of raw metal and sediment during the course of our lifetimes! The problem is that the human body cannot use the majority of these inorganic materials in our tap water.

For this reason, I recommend high-quality water filters that use either distillation or reverse osmosis.

#52 Liquid Sugar

One of the best ways to expand your fat cells, prematurely age your body, and erode your health potential is to down a soft drink loaded with sugar, caffeine, and phosphorous. The average soft drink contains about 10 teaspoons of sugar—that's 10 times more sugar than your body is programmed to handle at any one time. The National Soft Drink Association in the United States (yes, there is such an organization) reports that the average American guzzles back slightly more than 52 gallons of carbonated soft drinks per person per year (that's thousands of teaspoons of sugar). In fact, if you were to consume an average 12-ounce (360 ml) can of soda pop, you would be delivering almost 40 grams—or 10 teaspoons—of refined sugars to your body (yummy!).

Given these numbers, it's easy to see why so many of us are in hormonal havoc these days. The pop we drink elevates our insulin levels through the roof, enhancing our fat cell expansion (weight gain), and making us feel lousy from both a physiological and psychological standpoint.

#53 The Artificial Stuff

The artificial sweeteners found in many diet soft drinks, can affect your health just as negatively as sugar (and in some cases even more so). Sugar substitutes didn't exist when our bodies were evolving over thousands of years. Our bodies don't know what to do with them other than treat them as a type of sugar. Laboratory tests confirm that artificial sweeteners can boost our metabolic storage hormone insulin by fooling the body into thinking the sweetener is sugar and stimulating sugar cravings. When insulin can't find any real sugar from these substitutes, the insulin ends up going after our blood sugar, causing us to experience an energy decline and a fat-storage increase.

One study published in the *International Journal of Obesity* even showed that artificial sweeteners may actually enhance your desire to overeat by hindering your body's ability to estimate overall calorie intake, and in his ground-breaking book *Aspartame (NutraSweet) Is it Safe?* (Charles Press, 1992), Dr. Hyman Roberts states, "The American Cancer Society (1986) documented the fact that persons using artificial sweeteners gain more weight than those who avoid them."

#54 Magnesium and Water

Minerals, especially magnesium, are an essential part of a healthy metabolism. In fact, magnesium is essential to the maintenance of proper blood sugar levels and is required in more than 300 biochemical reactions—involved in every step the body uses to produce energy (ATP). Having said this, research presented in the *American Journal of the Collage of Nutrition* indicates that an alarming 19 percent of Americans don't even consume half of the recommended daily intake of 420 mg.

The fact remains that most bottled water and almost all tap water is void of this essential mineral (not to mention numerous other important ones) and studies indicate that communities with low levels of magnesium in their drinking water have an increased rate of sudden death. This "sudden death" may be due to the extensive role magnesium plays in both cardiovascular and metabolic health. After examining numerous studies on the association between cardiovascular death and water "hardness" (largely measured by magnesium and calcium levels), the World Health Organization (WHO) concluded that the lower the magnesium content in drinking water, the higher is the risk for cardiovascular disease, which means magnesium would probably be a great supplement to add to your Losing Fat 4 Life protocol.

How Much Water?

Health experts are still not 100 percent certain regarding exactly how much water is needed by the average person on a day-to-day basis—due to factors including amount of exercise, heat loss, illness, etc.—but the general consensus is that adults require anywhere from three-quarters to one ounce of water per pound of body weight. In other words, the average 120-pound woman should drink at least eight 8-ounce glasses of fluid per day. Drink the water in a closed container through a straw to avoid excess air and try squeezing a quarter of a lemon in your water if you find water too bland on its own.

CHAPTER 7

PROTEIN AND YOUR METABOLISM

Protein is absolutely essential for life. It helps increase your metabolic rate by creating an enhanced hormonal cascade essential for fat loss. Protein is second only to water as the most plentiful substance in the body. In fact, more than 50 percent of your body's dry weight is protein. The proteins you consume from the foods you eat are made up of subunits called amino acids.

Protein synthesis is the creation of new proteins from simple amino acids. It is one of our most vital anabolic processes. When we are young and vital, protein synthesis runs very efficiently, so we are predominantly anabolic. But as we age, our catabolic metabolism begins to exceed our anabolic metabolism, and the body's ability to construct protein starts to slow down. This is one of the reasons we lose muscle tissue and gain body fat with advancing age. Regular aging, excess stress and dieting causes a decline in protein synthesis and inevitably leads to a less than adequate metabolism for burning fat. The good news is that almost anyone has the ability to enhance their metabolism to more youthful levels, given the proper quality and amount of protein.

#55 The Metabolic Dance

As you are now aware, your body is in a constant battle between two opposing forces. The first force is anabolic, which is the process of body renewal. The second force is catabolic, which is the process of body breakdown. When your catabolic force overrides your anabolic force, you begin to break down on a cellular level and your metabolism rapidly declines. In other words, if you break down faster than your body can repair itself, you are in for quite a rough ride.

This elegant dance between *catabolism* and *anabolism* is one of the key factors to sustaining life. Every minute of every day, your body rebuilds, replaces, and replenishes about 200 million cells — that's almost 300 billion new cells by the time you wake up in the morning. The raw materials your body uses for this function are amino acids—found only in protein-containing foods. Carbohydrates can supply energy for building these body proteins, but they don't supply the actual raw building materials—only protein and certain fats can do that.

#56 Increasing Metabolism With Protein

High quality proteins consumed at regular intervals throughout the day help to increase your level of alertness all the while working to elevate your resting metabolic rate—even while you sleep. Compared with a high-carbohydrate meal, the thermogenic response (that is, the energy/heat produced) from a high-protein meal can be 40 percent greater. That's a lot of heat, and increased heat means more calories are burned.

Protein is also the main stimulator of the fat-burning hormone glucagon, which works opposite to the storage hormone insulin, allowing fat to be utilized as a fuel source instead of being used as extra padding. Research shows that protein meals increase oxygen consumption by two to three times more than a high-carbohydrate meal, indicating a much greater increase in the metabolic rate.

#57 Prehistoric Protein

We're not only what we eat, we are also what our ancestors ate. And guess what? Our ancestors ate lots of dietary proteins. According to medical anthropologist Dr. Boyd Eaton (who I referred to at the beginning of Chapter 1), our early diet consisted of at least 30 percent protein. Of course, the protein our ancestors ate was a little different from much of the protein we consume today. Early humans consumed protein from lean game meats that also contained the essential fatty acids that are often lacking in our diets today (more on this in the next chapter).

Other research indicates that we were predominantly hunters and then gatherers, but our ancestors had the same genes we have today. Our early ancestors were in some ways much healthier than the carbohydrate-loving, grain-fed humans of the agricultural revolution. According to case studies of prehistoric populations, these hunter-gatherers were tall, lean, muscular, strong, had dense bones, very little tooth decay (if any), and experienced very little disease.

#58 All Protein is Not Created Equal

The actual value of the various dietary protein foods is measured in something called a Net Protein Utilization (NPU) Index, which reflects the biological value, expressed as a percentage of digestibility of a specific dietary protein. The biological value of dietary protein is the efficiency with which that protein deposits the proper proportions and amounts of the essential amino acids needed for the building of body proteins. The important factor is not the amount of dietary protein consumed, but the amount of dietary protein that is available to the body after ingestion. And, the better the quality of protein you consume, the faster the results will show up on your new physique.

Our bodies all have their own specific amino acid profile, and there is no one food that fits that profile exactly. Other than the dietary protein found in our own mother's milk (perfect protein), all other proteins are rated in the NPU against the next best thing: an egg. The only food that has a higher NPU than whole eggs is properly filtered whey protein, but since whey protein is an engineered food of sorts, the egg remains the benchmark.

#59 Consuming Higher Quality Protein

If you consume only proteins that have a low biological value, then your body will have a much harder time utilizing the protein for structural (muscle, bone, organs, etc.) and functional (enzymes, neurotransmitters, hormones, etc.) goods. Protein can also be broken down as an energy source by the body. The problem is that when protein is burned for energy, it creates metabolic waste products in the form of ammonia. These nitrogenous waste products can overload the kidneys and liver, causing potential problems in people susceptible to kidney and liver ailments.

It is my opinion that the higher the quality of protein consumed, the more effectively that protein will be utilized for the important functions the body needs it for. Your body has plenty of fat and sugar to burn as fuel. You don't need to create extra waste for elimination by burning protein. It is better to consume smaller quantities of higher-quality proteins.

Animal vs. Vegetarian Proteins

Most of the dietary proteins we eat should come from foods such as lean cuts of—preferably grass-fed and organic—meats (venison, tenderloin, lamb), skinless poultry (free range: chicken breast, turkey breast, duck, ostrich, goose and quail), fish (always wild/never farmed: salmon, cod, tuna, bass, halibut, snapper, swordfish, trout, haddock and sole), seafood, some low-fat (organic only) dairy products like cottage cheese and plain yogurt (only if you are not sensitive to dairy), eggs and supplemental proteins derived from high-alpha whey protein (a minimum of 30 percent of the whey should be from alphalactalbumin, so read the label), sprouted brown rice and Moringa. No matter what the source, be a smart consumer and buy foods that are as fresh, organic, and free range as possible.

Plant-based dietary proteins, aside from sprouted brown rice, Moringa and hemp (preferably in that order) are very low in biological value. A sizable portion of dietary proteins from vegetables is never absorbed because the fiber in these foods binds to the protein. (The only exception to low NPU ratings when it comes to vegetable proteins are the ones listed above.) Active vegans, who only consume 100 percent plant-based foods, have one heck of a time building and repairing muscle tissue and maintaining an optimal metabolism. Many vegetable proteins are not only low in biological value (in terms of bioavailability) but also high in carbohydrates (particularly vegetables like beans, peas, and corn).

#60 The Best Whey to Support Metabolism

Whey is a by-product of the cheese-making process. Whey was actually regarded as waste until scientists researched the profiles of its chemical protein structure and decided to try to extract that protein. Early whey protein products were referred to as whey concentrates. They contained as little as 30 percent to 40 percent dietary proteins and were filled instead with huge amounts of fat, lactose (milk sugar), and denatured (damaged) proteins. The newest generation of whey isolates can contain more than 90 percent pure dietary proteins, with almost no dietary fats and minimal levels of lactose. They are also very expensive to produce. Due to the increased cost of the newer isolates, many manufacturers tend to mix the isolates with less expensive concentrates and still call them isolates. Only a very small percentage of companies use 100 percent isolates.

These proteins are extremely anabolic and are able to increase protein synthesis faster and better than other dietary proteins. Their superior amino acid profile gives them the edge over other dietary proteins when it comes to their digestibility and incorporation into muscle tissue. The protein also aids fat burning and muscle growth, works as an appetite suppressant, and can be used by those who are lactose intolerant, but make sure whatever whey protein you choose, it is not loaded with artificial sweeteners and flavoring agents.

#61 Wake Up with Protein

Normally, high protein containing meals tend to stimulate the brain, rather than sedate it—which is a great thing in the morning when you require more energy. Researchers have discovered a few main reasons for this. First off, complete proteins (like chicken, fish, eggs, whey) contain high levels of the amino acids *phenylalanine* and *tyrosine*, the building blocks of the brain-stimulating chemicals *dopamine* and *norepinephrine*. It is important to note that these proteins (along with three others) compete with tryptophan for entry into the brain, and more often than not win entry to help you feel more alert.

Not all proteins can elevate brain serotonin levels—especially in the evening. A double-blind, placebo-controlled study published in the *American Journal of Clinical Nutrition* indicated that whey protein containing high levels of alpha-lactalbumin, the exact kind found in my High-Alpha Whey Protein, could greatly increase plasma tryptophan levels in highly stressed individuals. High alpha-whey protein powders, then, are not only another great source of tryptophan, but also provide a way to make sure it gets into the brain to manufacture more serotonin.

#62 How Much Protein?

According to the Recommended Dietary Allowances (RDA) set out in Canada and the U.S. for dietary proteins, we shouldn't be taking in any more than 0.8 gram of protein per kilogram of body weight. While this amount may be acceptable for people who never move (there is actually a statement in the U.S.

RDA Handbook that reads, "In view of the margin of safety in the RDA no increment is added for work or training."), many researchers (including myself) believe that it is much too low for someone who wishes to gain muscle and support metabolism.

This certainly does not mean that you should over consume dietary proteins at any one sitting—too much protein in one meal can stress the liver and kidneys. The upper limit, depending on body size and activity level, seems to be 25 to 40 grams, or approximately 6 ounces, at one sitting. Obviously, this is just a general outline and is not intended to be an exact calculation (women need less protein than men and athletes need more protein than sedentary people, etc.)

#63 Protein Deficiency

We're all biochemically different and therefore our dietary protein requirements are different. Just assume that the more active you are, the more dietary protein you will need to repair the body. Dr. Lee Coyne points out in his book <u>Fat Won't Make You Fat</u> that according to some of the most respected researchers in the field of nutrition, the RDAs for dietary proteins can be low by at least a factor of three. This assertion is further backed by research by Dr. Emanuel Cheraskin, formerly from the University of Alabama. After assessing the Cornell Medical Index Health Questionnaire filled out by 1,040 dentists and their spouses, Dr. Cheraskin found that those who consumed two to three times the RDA of dietary proteins had the fewest medical health problems.

Individual dietary protein intake and absorption is also affected by the way the proteins are prepared and the accessory nutrients that are available for the assimilation of the proteins. Dietary proteins require a full array of the B vitamins in order to be properly utilized and incorporated into body tissues, so make sure you are supplementing with adequate B vitamins.

Add a Protein Shake or Two

High-Alpha Whey Protein is nature's best source of complete protein and is an excellent anabolic enhancer. It has also been scientifically proven to offer many other health-enhancing benefits, such as increased antioxidant protection, hunger control, increased metabolism, increased brain function, cancer prevention and heart disease prevention. This is why I have recommended making two protein shakes a day (preferably with High-Alpha Whey Protein) for over 10 years now.

CHAPTER 8

CARBS AND YOUR METABOLISM

No word strikes fear into a person who is trying to lose fat than the word carbohydrate, but the truth is not all carbohydrates are our enemy and it is imperative to understand that some components of carbohydrates actually help us lose fat... yes, you read that right, some carbohydrates help us to lose fat.

But first, what is a carbohydrate? Carbohydrates come mainly from plants—which include grains, vegetables, and fruits. Refined or processed carbohydrates also exist, such as flour and sugar, which have become the staples of our diets throughout North America. Refined carbs are also a big reason we are experiencing our obesity epidemic.

#64 Carbohydrates = Sugar

In order for foods to become usable substances in the body, their matter must first be broken down into its simplest form. In the case of carbohydrates, they are broken down into simple sugars like glucose—each carbohydrate food has an equivalent expressed as sugar. It's very important for you to realize that all carbohydrates eventually break down into sugar in the body. Whether you consume one-fourth cup of pure sugar or eat a baked potato, in the end they both become one-fourth cup of sugar to your body and your body will take the appropriate steps to bring its new sugar levels back into balance.

Does this mean that a baked potato is as bad for you as one-fourth cup of sugar? Of course not. But, in terms of your battle of the bulge, you must realize that your body can only deal with so much sugar at a time (One teaspoon). Any excess will wreak havoc on your hormonal systems. Winning your fat war is all about balance.

#65 Carbohydrates and Insulin

I touched on this briefly in Chapter 1, but I feel it is far too elaborate on the carbohydrate/insulin connection here as well. Refined carbohydrates (and sugars) raise blood glucose levels quickly and are the biggest contributors to high insulin levels and elevated insulin levels are an over-fat person's nightmare. The body can't access fat as a fuel source when there are high levels of insulin floating around. And a very large percentage of people—especially over-fat people—have high resting insulin levels most, if not all, of the time. In fact, over-fat people have high insulin levels not only in their blood, but also in their cells, creating a sluggish metabolism.

The overflow of insulin has been proven to spell the end to fat loss goals and, in the process, cause a lot of destruction. In a 1996 experiment, people were given substances to increase their insulin and blood-sugar levels, plus an infusion of various fatty acids. The experiment showed that both glucose and insulin determine how effectively fat gets burned as fuel: high glucose/insulin levels reduced the concentration of the enzyme that transports fatty acids for burning to 45 percent of its normal level.

#66 Should You Avoid a High-Carbohydrate Diet?

A high-carbohydrate diet creates a vicious circle. At the muscle cell level, years of poor diet, likely combined with a lack of exercise and stress, cause muscle cells to go flat. Over-carbed and under-worked muscle cells just don't function as they should—they're like a stagnant pond that's practically devoid of life. So not only is there an oversupply of blood sugar, but it also can't get into the flat muscle cell; it's floating around in the bloodstream with no place to go.

An alarm rings out in the pancreas: pump out more insulin—NOW! For hours, perhaps all day, insulin is elevated to deal with this blood sugar onslaught. As you are now well aware, this stops fat burning cold. In fact, it jams a great amount of the meal right into your billions of waiting fat cells. You know the saying, "Might as well apply it directly to my hips"? Nothing burned, everything gained. Some of the worst offenders happen to come from processed breads, white rice and pasta.

#67 The Glycemic Index

Many carbohydrate-rich foods are ranked according to how fast they get into the bloodstream, on a scale from 0 to 100 called the *glycemic index*. The index measures the speed at which the carbohydrates break down and put sugar into the bloodstream. Some break down quickly during digestion, causing a drastic rise in blood sugar levels. These have the highest glycemic index rating. Glucose, at a dose of 50 grams, is used as the benchmark and is given a rating of 100 because it raises blood sugar super fast. Other carbohydrates are ranked in relation to glucose. The glycemic index measures how much your blood glucose increases over a period of two or three hours after a meal.

Dr. David Jenkins, professor of nutrition at the University of Toronto, was the first to develop the concept of the glycemic index to help determine which foods are best suited for people with blood sugar disorders (diabetes). In 1981, Dr. Jenkins released a groundbreaking study called *"Glycemic Index of Foods: A Physiological Basis for Carbohydrate Exchange"*. In the subsequent years, hundreds of clinical studies in the United Kingdom, France, Italy, Canada, and Australia have proved the value of the glycemic index. To find out where your favorite foods fall, visit: www.glycemicindex.com.

> **Keeping Blood Sugar Low**
>
> One trick to keeping blood sugar low and insulin in check is to eat like a caveman. That is, eat like we did when all we had access to, were natural, unprocessed foods. The foods at the bottom of the food chain—the unprocessed fruits (especially from the berry family) and vegetables that are high in fiber and water—are among the lowest on the glycemic index. In contrast, highly processed foods—the ones we either "improved" or that are completely artificial—like white pasta and breads are among the highest.

#68 Fiber the Good Carbohydrate

Fiber is technically a carbohydrate, with the exception that your body can't digest it. It is also one of those macronutrients that seems to get lost in the shuffle. For most people the word fiber means bland tasting foods like bran. But the truth is that fiber does not have to be bland at all, in fact, once you understand how important fiber is to your metabolic success you won't ever want to be without it again.

Nutritional researchers have known for years that dietary fiber contributes to the reduction of excess body fat, high blood sugar and high cholesterol. It also lowers the glycemic value of a food and promotes health of the bowel by providing a mild cleansing effect. The latter effect ultimately has the ability to result in any number of preventive health benefits. The problem is that the great majority of our population doesn't get enough fiber in their diet.

#69 Losing Fat with Fiber

The reason dietary fiber is so important, is because the right fibers can greatly increase the body's ability to remove excess fat by lowering excess insulin. Research presented in the *International Journal of Obesity* indicates that an increased intake of dietary fiber is useful for the treatment of both obesity and *diabetes mellitus*. Fiber accomplishes its insulin-modulating/fat loss effects by slowing the release of sugars into the bloodstream—thereby preventing a high surge of insulin—and upgrading insulin sensitivity—especially within the muscle cells. When insulin receptors are activated in muscle cells, there is correspondingly low insulin receptor activity in the fat cells, making it extremely difficult for your fat cells to expand.

Studies have shown that adding 5 to 30 grams of fiber (especially gel-forming ones like oat beta glucan and guar gum found in the 100 percent food-derived organic FibreLean formula) per day to a healthy diet leads to an increased sense of fullness, which ultimately reduces the desire to consume extra calories that contribute to body fat stores.

#70 Soluble, Insoluble—What Does It All Mean?

Most people know that there are two main forms of fiber, soluble and insoluble, but the fact remains that understanding what each one is beneficial for can get a little confusing. This confusion—between the amounts of soluble and insoluble fiber needed in the diet—has led a National Academy of Sciences Panel to recommend that the terms "soluble and insoluble" fibers gradually be eliminated and replaced by specific beneficial physiological effects of fiber (phew!).

The take-home message is: it is more important to concentrate on the overall intake of <u>any</u> and <u>all</u> fibers, than it is to concern yourself with consuming a specific variety. The point is that all natural fiber contributes to overall health in one way or another—especially those derived by vegetables (green leafy ones) and fruits (like berries).

#71 How Much Fiber?

In May 2001, the prestigious National Academy of Sciences released a comprehensive report on fiber as a part of their multi-year study on dietary reference intakes. Its report concluded that the recommended amount of fiber that should be included in the daily human diet, a minimum of **35 grams a day**, is considerably higher than what most individuals will consume, or can reasonably be expected to consume based upon today's average diet (which happens to include a measly 10-15 grams of fiber on average).

In fact, our hunter-gatherer brothers and sisters ate almost 100 grams of fiber a day. That's six to ten times what we consume today!

Metabolism-supporting fibers

The following are a few of the most research-proven metabolism-supporting fibers and what they help achieve:

Inulin (FOS): Is classified as a prebiotic—a nutrient that is fermented in the large bowel that enhances the growth of desirable bacteria or microflora. Prebiotics provide many of the same positive benefits of soluble fiber with the addition of being able to modulate various areas of the immune system. This enhanced immunity is achieved through direct contact of lactic acid bacteria with immune cells in the intestine and the production of short-chain fatty acids from fiber fermentation. Inulin also provides an enhanced bioavailability of essential minerals—especially magnesium—and supplies a good source of calcium, vitamin A and potassium.

Guar gum: Is a great source of soluble fiber derived from the seed of the guar bean, a plant native to India. According to research, guar gum has been shown to prevent blood sugar increases after ingesting sweetened foods, delay the absorption of sugars from the intestines, exert a beneficial effect on bowel management, and increase the satiety (fullness) hormone CCK. It is also proven to act as a prebiotic to aid in beneficial bacteria counts in the intestine.

Oat beta glucan: Is one of nature's richest sources of soluble fiber found within oat bran. Beta-glucans have been shown to help lower serum cholesterol, aid in proper insulin control and stimulate immunity. Oat beta glucans contain high levels of tocotrienols—antioxidants that are part of the Vitamin E family, but contain many times more antioxidant potential.

#72 Alert or Sleepy?

Have you ever wondered why certain meals make youfeel great, while others leave you feeling sluggish and ready to hit the sack? The answer lies within the way various nutrients from these foods interact with various brain chemicals that work to either enhance our levels of alertness and motivation or make us feel tired and sleepy.

Nutritionists have always known that meals comprised primarily of improper carbohydrates (i.e., fiber-void carbs like white bread) can cause us to feel less than energetic, while meals high in protein can help us feel alert.

CHAPTER 9

FAT AND YOUR METABOLISM

Contrary to popular belief, dietary fats (fatty acids) don't always make us fat. In fact, some fats actually help us lose unwanted body fat. Over the last 30 years or so, we have seen low-fat diets hit the market in a big way, leading us to believe that if we replaced fat-laden foods with low-fat (or no-fat) foods, our problems would be solved. Because dietary fat has nine calories per gram, compared with 4 calories per gram of carbs, we assumed that if we just reduced our consumption of dietary fats and raised our consumption of carbohydrates, we would lose fat. As you are now aware, this is far from the case.

#73 Low-Fat Diets are Actually High-Carbohydrate Diets in Disguise

Rule #1, fat consumption is essential to the functioning of your body—especially where your metabolism is concerned. It's just that the wrong type of dietary fats can turn muscle cells into lousy fat burners. Many research studies show that if we keep our "good" dietary fat consumption within the range of 20 percent to 35 percent of total food intake, there is no worry of becoming fat. In fact, as you will find out in this chapter, we can't live without fat. Even prestigious organizations such as the Canadian Heart and Stroke Foundation and the American Heart Association now suggest that we should be consuming up to 30 percent of our calories from the right types of fats (more on this later).

Too many people have tried cutting all the fat from their diets, only to find, to their amazement, that instead of the fat magically disappearing, they had an even harder time losing it. It is this unwarranted fear of fats or "fat phobia" that has led to our overwhelming carbohydrate indulgence of the last 20 years. When you restrict fat intake, not only do you limit beneficial fatty acids that are needed by every cell of the body, but you end up restoring the caloric deficit with extra carbohydrates (usually of the high-glycemic variety). Therefore, most low-fat diets are actually high-carbohydrate diets in disguise.

#74 Cutting the Fat

What really happens to your body when you decide to cut out most of the fats from your diet and replace them with extra carbohydrates? This question was answered during a study at Rockefeller University in New York. Normal-weight people were placed on either a 40 percent fat diet or a 10 percent fat diet and checked every 10 days to see how much fat they were making. Yes, the body is very good at *making* fat from carbohydrates.

Those on the high-fat diet were making little or no fat, as measured by triglyceride levels and triglyceride content. Those on the low-fat diet, however, were having a very different reaction. Doctors discovered that between 30 percent and 57 percent of the fatty acids in the bloodstream was saturated fat manufactured by the body. In short, those eating low-fat, high-carbohydrate diets made more of their own saturated fat!

Genetically, we haven't changed much from thousands of years ago when we consumed wild game, fish, and nuts. How were these foods different from the foods of today? Not only were they low glycemic, but they also contained good amounts of friendly fats. Today, our diets have a totally different dietary-fat content from the ones we were genetically made for, which is why we suffer from many unfriendly fat-related diseases, including cardiovascular disease, arthritis, diabetes, hypertension, and obesity, just to name a few.

#75 Separating the Fat

Dietary fats are essential to life: it's the type of fat you eat that can make all the difference in the world. Natural whole foods contain dietary fats as part of their structural components, and have a balance of *saturated* fats, *monounsaturated* fats, and *polyunsaturated* fats. The wrong fats, like trans fats, or *too much* saturated fat from animal products, can cause your fat-burning muscle cells to become sluggish and lazy.

A saturated fat is simply a dietary fat with no hydrogen vacancies. This means that the carbon chain is carrying its maximum number of hydrogen atoms. These fats are vital to our biochemistry, but our bodies can usually manufacture all that they need from raw materials (food). Saturated fats have a molecularly straight structure that allows them easy access into our already bulging fat cells (like arrows entering a bull's-eye). In essence, they are only useful as fuel, and no one has to remind us of how much extra fuel we are already carrying. They are found in high concentrations in meat and dairy products. In *excess*, they contribute to obesity, cardiovascular disease, certain cancers, and insulin insensitivity.

#76 Not All Saturated Fats are Bad

To set the record straight, it is important to note that not all saturated fats are the bad guys we've been led to believe. Dr. Mary Enig, one of the foremost experts on fats and oils, has done extensive research in this area, and found that the consumption of animal fat has actually decreased from 83 percent of total fat consumption to 53 percent in the North American diet over the last 80 years. In this same time, vegetable fat consumption has jumped from 17 percent to 47 percent.

It is Dr. Enig's belief that this rise in consumption of vegetable fat is correlated with the rise in cancer and possibly obesity. But the vegetable fat that Dr. Enig and many other fatty-acid researchers are most concerned with is the unnatural trans fats from *hydrogenated* and *partially hydrogenated* oils. Trans fat is found in commercially available baked goods like bread, crackers, chips, cookies, pies, and doughnuts.

#77 Frankenstein of the Fats

"Frankenstein fats" is one name for the artificially altered fats that are more often called trans fats. Trans fats include those fats found in fried foods, margarine, and most bakery products. Trans fats have been chemically transformed through heat and hydrogenation (the process of filling in vacancies on the carbon chain by adding hydrogen atoms). By adding hydrogen atoms and altering the structures of healthy essential fats, food scientists give these fats longer shelf lives. Good for business, bad for health.

By hydrogenating these once-healthy, biologically active fats, we alter them in such a way that they become even more easily incorporated into our cellular membranes. This quirk in our biochemistry causes much confusion at the cellular level, leading to a leaking effect in our cellular membranes and ultimately causing chaos with many biochemical functions, including the closing down of our fat-burning machinery. Trans fats have also been shown to increase insulin, decrease testosterone, reduce energy metabolism, increase bad cholesterol, and inhibit immune function, just to name a few of the side effects.

#78 What Are You Made Of?

Typically, in Western industrialized nations, human fat cells store more than

50 percent monounsaturated fatty acids, 30 percent to 40 percent saturated fatty acids, and 10 percent to 20 percent polyunsaturates. This is a reflection of the ratio of dietary fats we consume. Among the polyunsaturates in fat-cell triglycerides, less than one percent is from the omega-3 family. This means we're very much omega-3 deficient. Since 1850, omega-3 consumption has decreased to one-sixth its traditional (healthy) level, resulting in an omega-6 to omega-3 ratio of 20:1, with an optimum ratio being between 1:1 for the brain and 4:1 for the lean tissues.

High levels of omega-6 EFAs as a whole suppress the uptake of omega-3s into tissues. By increasing the amount of omega-3 essential fatty acids in our diet with foods like hempseed, flaxseed oil and cold-water fish (containing EPA and DHA), we'll be able to reintroduce this important class of nutrients into our cells.

#79 Not Just Good Fats—They're Essential

Omega-6—known as *linoleic acid* or LA (which comes primarily from vegetable oils, animal fats, eggs and milk products) and Omega-3—known as *alpha-linolenic acid* or ALA (coming from hempseed, flaxseed, coldwater fish and krill), are classed as *essential fatty acids* (EFAs). These dietary fats are different from other fats because the body cannot manufacture them; they must be consumed. They are both polyunsaturated.

These two fats are considered essential because they supply the building blocks of various structures within the body. These include the cell membranes that enclose every one of our 100 trillion cells and the raw ingredients in the structures of eyes, ears, the brain, sex glands, and adrenal glands. EFAs also regulate the traffic of substances in and out of our cells, keeping foreign molecules, viruses, yeasts, fungi, and bacteria outside of cells, and keeping cell proteins, enzymes, genetic material, and organelles (like the mitochondria where fat is burned) inside the cells.

#80 The Messengers of Fat Burning

Omega-6s and omega-3s are precursors to a biologically powerful group of hormone-like messengers called *eicosanoids*. Eicosanoids are continuously produced (in minute quantities) in our cells, existing for less than a few seconds. They affect nearly every biochemical process in the body. The group of eicosanoids that are directly involved in fat metabolism are called *prostaglandins* (PGs). The E series of PGs are the ones most important to fat tissue regulation.

It is of the utmost importance to note that all prostaglandins are important regulators of our biochemistry. However, when we produce excess amounts of the PGE-2 series, things get a little out of whack. When in excess (as is typically the case among North Americans), PGE-

2s can be viewed as bad guys due to the powerful inflammatory potential they possess. In reality, we need this prostaglandin for many vital functions. The problem arises when the system is out of balance, when there is too much activity in this family. An imbalance of this prostaglandin can also be detrimental to your fat-burning efforts.

PGEs and the Foods They Come From

PGE-1Series:

Sunflower, safflower, sesame, and corn oils; primrose, borage, and blackcurrant seed oils

PGE-2Series:

Animal meat, milk, eggs, squid, warm water fish

PGE-3Series:

Moringa, flax, hemp, pumpkin, chia, walnut, brazil nut, cold-water fish, krill, and algae (some)

---

81 Bring on the Monounsaturates

Monounsaturated fats (MUFA) are important to overall health, especially when the goals are low blood triglyceride, low LDL cholesterol, and low glucose levels. A high consumption of MUFA contributes to a lower incidence of cardiovascular disease and diabetes. MUFAs also act as antioxidants, reducing the free radicals produced by LDL cholesterol oxidation. Research on people with diabetes has shown that a diet high in MUFA can reduce blood levels of triglycerides by 19 percent, LDL cholesterol by 14 percent, and VLDL cholesterol by 22 percent. That's a sizable decrease considering that many lipid and cholesterol-lowering drugs don't deliver these kinds of results, and carry with them serious side effects.

Oils rich in MUFAs include olive, avocado, walnut, canola, and high-oleic safflower oil. They're a great addition to our arsenal of fat-fighting weapons. Mediterranean diets are high in MUFAs because of the high amount of olive oil consumed. In fact, Mediterranean people consume up to 40 percent of their calories as fat and still have some of the lowest incidences of heart disease in the world today. MUFAs are also great at supporting a healthy metabolism, so be sure to make them the premier fat in your diet.

Fat with Carbs: The Deadly Duo

Fat requires both high levels of an enzyme called *lipoprotein lipase* (LPL) and high insulin levels in order to be stored within your billions of fat cells. In the absence of LPL and insulin, dietary fat will have a very hard time ending up in your fat cells. Unfortunately, when dietary fat is consumed along with high-glycemic carbohydrates, then most of the fat and additional sugars from the carbs become stored body fat.

The reason for this is because insulin—stimulated from the carbs—turns on the LPL enzyme, making it very easy to store fat. Foods such as ice cream or potato chips that contain a lot of fat along with sugars are excellent combinations if you want to increase your waist size in a hurry. The sugar in these foods (yes, even from the broken-down starch from the potato chips) boosts your insulin and LPL levels, and the fat from these foods gets shuttled into your eagerly waiting fat cells straightaway.

CHAPTER 10

DON'T EXERCISE— BIOCIZE™

Throughout much of the late twentieth-century, we North Americans have come face-to-face with a unique disease called *hypokinesis* that carries with it devastating consequences. Hypokinesis is just a fancy way of saying, "we suffer from too little bodily movement." Simply stated, "Your body is designed to move," and if you continue to practice a life of lethargy, you shouldn't be surprised when later on in life you are greeted with a fatter energy-deprived body! Studies confirm that reductions in activity levels are strongly correlated with increases in body fat, even when your calorie intake is significantly reduced—which is why you should never follow a diet without a proper exercise program.

Proper exercise which I define as Biocize™ helps create an optimum metabolic environment for continual fat release all day long. By incorporating Biocize strategies with the eating principles outline in this book, you can't help but create a metabolism that is primed for fat burning.

#82 Do You Really Have to Exercise?

No one would argue the point that exercise is something the vast majority of our population would rather avoid—like the plague—than engage in on a regular basis. But the truth remains that avoiding regular exercise—if your goal is to lead a healthy lean life—IS NOT AN OPTION! If you are truly serious about awakening your body to lose fat for life, then you will need to adopt a different outlook on exercise—one that actually finds you looking forward to it!

The number one reason most people don't stick to an exercise program long enough to see the results they have dreamed about, is because of their negative attitudes towards the exercise. Let's be honest, if you simply don't like something, you're not exactly going to look forward to it, and you will make all sorts of excuses to avoid it—as often as possible. But if your negative attitude towards whatever it was you don't like suddenly turned into a positive outlook, perhaps even one of excitement, you would actually embrace and even crave this new feeling. Yes, even for exercise.

#83 Say No to Sarcopenia

By the time of retirement age, the average sedentary North American will lose anywhere from one-third to one-half of their lean body mass and gain the rest in body fat. A metaphor I often use in my lectures is, "We seem to go from firm young Macintosh apples to soft mushy ones." We may weigh the same at retirement age as we did in our twenties, but things definitely look and feel different. We in a sense, become smaller, fatter people.

This age-related loss of muscle has been named *sarcopenia*, from the Greek for "flesh reduction." You don't hear a lot about sarcopenia in the news because most of its debilitating end effects are seen as *osteoporosis* or the loss of skeletal mass, and osteoporosis is what gets all the attention. The fact is that muscular contractions are needed to help keep your bones strong, and any loss of muscle tissue ultimately equates to weaker bones.

#84 Sarcopenia is Rampant

Due to our widespread distaste for regular proper exercise, sarcopenia has become rampant in our society.

According to Dr. William Evans, director of the nutrition, metabolism, and exercise lab at the University of Arkansas for Medical Sciences, "Nursing homes are filled with elderly people who are institutionalized not because of any disease or cognitive impairment, but because of muscle weakness." The only reason sarcopenia has been overlooked until now, is because muscle loss and weakness was considered yet another inevitable part of getting older. But, much research has proven otherwise.

Numerous studies demonstrate that proper exercise can help people even in their eighties and nineties improve their overall muscle size and strength—often to the point where they no longer need any assistance to perform everyday tasks. In a 1990 ground-breaking study presented in the prestigious *Journal of the American Medical Association*, muscle size and strength was greatly improved in as little as eight weeks of weight training, even in 90-year-old subjects.

#85 The Only Weight That Matters

Muscle is the key metabolic engine of your body, and each cell is loaded with thousands of those tiny little powerhouse engines called mitochondria. When you allow your body to lose its muscle mass, you invariably end up losing the ability to burn more calories while at rest. One pound of muscle tissue can burn at least 50 extra calories throughout the day. Muscle loss is also one of the major reasons most people end up failing at diets.

When you constantly diet, your body ends up eating away at its own proteins (muscle tissue) to make up for the deficit of incoming protein. Since you have lost muscle mass, your body is no longer able to utilize the same number of incoming calories so the extra calories are deposited within your billions of fat cells, which is why many people experience the rebound effect of putting on extra pounds when they go back to eating the way they did before the diet.

#86 Throw Away the Bathroom Scale

So, as you now know, all weight is not created equal. This is why I tell people to throw away their bathroom scales and stop obsessing over "weight loss" and become interested in losing the only weight you need to get rid of—your excess body fat. The real question you or anyone else should be asking on any fat loss program should be, "If I'm losing weight, where are those pounds coming from?" For every pound of body fat most people lose on an unbalanced fad diet, they should also expect the loss of a pound of muscle tissue. If you allow yourself to lose the very substance needed to burn fat in the first place, do you really think you're ahead in the game? I think not!

Biocize or proper physical exercise doesn't mean hardcore sports or working out in a gym with excessively heavy weights. Instead, it can mean performing fun weight bearing (lifting weights) exercises and proper cardio (more on this in a bit) in a fitness center or <u>the privacy of your own home</u> two to four times a week and for only 30–45 minutes at a time.

#87 Don't Only Do Cardio

Studies show that excessive aerobic training can actually be harmful, especially when muscle becomes a scarce resource as you age. Too much aerobic training actually causes muscles to atrophy and only burns fat during the first few sessions. After that, your body ultimately adjusts to such a predictable routine and jogging may do nothing but make you a smaller fat person. The same can be said for walking. Like running, walking has been touted as some sort of magical fountain of fat loss; however, if it is your sole form of exercise, it's akin to bringing a squirt gun to the OK corral. Sure, walking should be part of any fit lifestyle, but if it is your only form of exercise, you can expect your two legs to be carrying around a skimpy, plump body for the better part of your life.

Allan Geliebter, PhD, and his colleagues at Columbia University recently put the tried and true wisdom that steady state aerobic exercise like jogging and diet helps people lose appreciable weight and fat. Over the course of eight weeks, those that dieted and did aerobics three times per week lost the same amount of fat and weight as those that simply cut calories. In other words, they wasted their time!

#88 Interval Training Is the New Cardio

Exercising the "right way" means chucking long running or walking sessions in the proverbial trashcan. Instead, adopt an entirely new and more effective cardio approach, known as interval- training. Interval-training is basically a higher intensity form of cardio done in a fraction of the time wasted on most cardio workouts. Dozens of studies have proven that interval-training burns more fat in less time.

Take this study that compared interval training with old-school cardio for 15-weeks. One group did 20 minutes of interval training three times per week. The other group spent 40 minutes three times per week on steady-state cardio work. Even though the interval-training group spent half as much time exercising, they lost six pounds of fat, while the steady state group actually *gained* fat. In other words, even though it eats up more time, steady state cardio created a group of smaller fat people.

#89 In Biocize—Synergy Is the Key

Along with interval training it is imperative to the success of your metabolism to perform regular (two to three times per week) bouts of resistance training (some interval classes incorporate resistance exercises into their programs) in order to increase lean body mass (muscle tissue) and strength. In fact, research shows that the combination of the two equals much greater results.

In a landmark study published in the *American Journal of Cardiology*, aerobic training was compared to aerobic with resistance (weight) training. Participants were split into two groups and had to complete a ten-week exercise program of 75 minutes. One group completed 75 minutes of aerobic exercise twice a week, while the other completed 40 minutes of aerobics plus 35 minutes of weight training. The time-spent training was identical. At the end of the study, the aerobics group presented an 11 percent increase in endurance, but no increase in their strength. The group that completed the combination of aerobics plus weight training showed a massive 109 percent increase in their endurance, and a 21 percent to 43 percent increase in their overall strength. There are many other studies that further prove the theory that resistant training with low impact cardio is superior to either one alone.

#90 Life Is Not Meant to be Lived In a Gym

The greatest effects of Biocize actually occur after the activity is completed—say what! This is due to a rise in anabolic (rebuild and repair) hormones, testosterone and growth hormone—approximately 15 minutes—after the exercise is completed. As long as you don't blunt this metabolic increase by consuming high-carbohydrate energy drinks in the absence of protein, your body will have the ability to burn calories for many hours to come.

In one study, it was shown that over two-thirds of the fat-burning activity of exercise takes place after the actual exercise sessions. This increase in fat burning potential has been documented as lasting for over 15 hours in highly trained athletes, and is believed to be due to the increased activity of the fat releasing enzyme, HSL.

CHAPTER 11

THE POWER OF BELIEF

I often say in my lectures that too many of us suffer from a condition called acceptance. We accept our excess body fat and our less then optimal health status as the way we are just meant to feel with each advancing year. How sad! We accept this as the truth, when in fact it is nothing but smoke and mirrors—an illusion. The reality however is it's our illusion and therefore our reality.

It is far easier for people to believe that living a lean life of energy and abundance is for the lucky ones... those that were born with the genes to embrace this life.... that being lean and healthy was never a life they were destined for. And for the majority, they also believe that having a coffee and a few donuts for breakfast, pizza for lunch and a hamburger and fries (and let's not forget Diet Coke) for dinner, won't make a difference in their life's path. Let's face it, if mom and pop are sporting an extra 50 to 100 pounds, then that must be your destiny too... right?

Absolutely not! We all have the ability to live a lean life of abundant energy; but unfortunately, we don't have the power of belief to make it happen. We are all meant to live life, but in order to live, one must be truly alive. This is why you must reawaken your body and your mind in order to experience what you have been missing for far too long—true life. This is where the power of belief comes in.

#90 What Is Your Present Reality?

My goal for this book is to guide you through to a new truth, a new reality, and one that ultimately becomes your very own. My wish is for you to finally experience true life! For you to adopt and practice the principles necessary to reawaken what lies deep within you, all you have to do is believe that it is possible, apply the principles outlined throughout this book and have the willpower to see it through to the end, or in this case, the beginning—of the new you!

I have never promised anyone that changing one's life—for the better—is an easy process, quite the opposite in fact. It is much easier to sit back and do nothing at all. Lethargy, lack of exercise, bad eating habits and all the other things the majority of North Americans are known for, are learned and practiced habits that eventually became a reality. The question is—what is your present reality?

"If you believe you can, you probably can. If you believe you won't, you most assuredly won't. Belief is the ignition switch that gets you off the launching pad."

—*Denis Waitley*

#91 Change Your Destiny

The late Dr. Maxwell Maltz, one of the most widely known and highly regarded plastic surgeons of our time explained in his mega bestselling book <u>Psycho-Cybernetics</u> (Psycho-Cybernetics Foundation), some patients—*no matter how physically-altered through surgery*—show no change at all in their personality. It's as if nothing at all changes, and that in their minds they still remained scarred or ugly. Dr. Maltz later went on to discover that a person's "self-image" or the true way in which the individual perceived themselves, became the real key to a person's personality and behavior, and ultimately their reality.

The key to success on any program is to remember that you are the one in control of your destiny—no one else! Change your old unhealthy habits for new healthy ones presented throughout this book and you will ultimately look, feel and perform better than you ever thought possible. Awakening your body and your true life's potential is a lot closer then you may presently believe!

#92 Self-Efficacy

Researchers at the University of Montreal wanted to see whether the action of believing in one's weight-loss success resulted in lower attrition rates. 62 women signed up for the study and were assessed on how confident they were that they'd lose the weight they wanted. After six months, the variable most tied to successful weight loss and continued participation was self-efficacy.

After surveying hundreds of overweight older women, Australian scientist Rhonda Anderson, PhD, has seen the potential for self-efficacy in overcoming inevitable obstacles: "Self-efficacy is our belief that we can produce the result we want to produce, so a person with high dietary self-efficacy believes they can eat healthily no matter what—even when bored, upset, tired, on holiday or at a party." Many other studies, including well-designed randomized control trials, have found that self-efficacy is especially important in weight maintenance—which is by far the most elusive and challenging aspect of any fat loss plan.

"Believe and act as if it were impossible to fail." —Charles F. Kettering

#93 Are You Subconsciously Holding Onto Your Fat?

Our actions are controlled by both the conscious and subconscious mind. Unfortunately, the subconscious mind—which developed long before our conscious mind did (as in the womb)—is about one million times more powerful a processor than the conscious mind is, so if it is filled with negative beliefs, we make these misperceptions our realities. The subconscious mind is like a tape recorder that can't be turned off. It plays in the background and acts without your permission. The only way to change the program is to rewrite it.

For most, it's the subconscious mind that derails fat loss attempts more than any reduced-fat cake could ever hope to do. Simply put, most people sabotage their fat loss success. Perhaps you chase after fad diets because you know they won't work. The fact that you regain all the weight you lost, and then some, might actually be because you aren't ready to deal with the real problems in your life. In other words, you aren't willing—or able—to shed the protective blanket you've become so comfortable snuggled up in all these years. Say what!

#94 Protecting Yourself with Fat

For those with a low sense of self-worth, obesity allows them to forgo close relationships to avoid rejection or emotional hurt. It's been documented in various studies that many people gain weight to prevent sexual or romantic advances and that this avoidance stems from fear of loss or as remnants of abuse. The weight is like a bodyguard keeping meaningful interpersonal attachment from getting in.

Perhaps you assume that weight is the only thing holding you back from health, wealth, and happiness. However, the subconscious mind realizes that your circumstances are the result of hundreds of mitigating factors—many of which have nothing to do with how much you weigh. This is why many people get depressed after losing weight. They realize that their hopes and dreams weren't dependent on one factor and they have to finally face the decisions they made that got them to where they are. It's a lot easier to point the blame at a single factor than to face reality.

#95 Emotional Eating

Why do we emotionally eat? A study published in Qualitative Health Research found that people's drive to emotionally eat is "not about the food." Even though sugary foods have a magnet-like attraction to painful emotions, the food itself isn't the driving force. In order to maintain the fat that's essential as a prop for our coping mechanism we have to eat more than our stomach tells us we require. But, emotional eating can also serve another important purpose: substituting as a loved one.

When psychologists study the emotions people experience after they've lost weight, a consistent theme is that many mourn the "loss of a friend." In some ways, food is more reliable than a loved one. It's not uncommon for overly fat people to project the values they look for in others onto food. Food is commonly referred to as "reliable," "comforting," and even "understanding"—all things we crave in the ones we love. When we lack emotional attachment, a lack of a social circle for example, we literally fill the emptiness we feel inside with food.

#96 Social Support and Personal Accountability

Brown University researchers took a set of people who recently lost 40 pounds and put them into three groups: one received a newsletter, another got internet support, while the third group met with a counselor face-to-face. They wanted to see which method would help keep the weight from piling back on, as it always seems to do. Over the course of a year and a half, the group that met with a real person regained less than half the weight (and just five pounds).

Another study, this one published in the *Journal of Consulting and Clinical Psychology* concluded that people who received typical weight-loss counseling along with support from a friend had a 40 percent better chance of keeping weight off than those that went at it alone. While some people have it out for us (and usually they are fighting their weight as well and are not ready to make the change themselves), more times than not, leaning on someone supportive helps keep the fat boomerang at bay.

#97 Keep With It No Matter What

People are notorious for reaching a small goal (of say losing 10 pounds) and then falling back into their old habits. The same ones that got them to the place they didn't need to be (i.e., over fat). The longer you stick with the program—in this case, your new lifestyle strategy—the easier it becomes to continue on your new path.

A study published in the journal, *Obesity Research,* showed that the longer people are successful at keeping excess weight off their frames, the easier it becomes and the less effort it requires as time goes by. This makes sense since the more a behavior—*such as exercising or eating right*—is repeated, the more likely it is to become a habit.

> *"You can have anything you want if you will give up the belief that you can't have it."* —Dr. Robert Anthony

#98 Belief and Exercise

If you plan to change the way you look, feel and perform, proper exercise is no longer an option. But unfortunately, 50 percent of the people that start an exercise program in the New Year, quit during the first six months. Could it be that the 50 percent who quit don't have enough self-belief? A study published in the *Journals of Gerontology* indicates that how you think (in terms of what exercise can or cannot do for you), will determine how well exercise will work for you.

After questioning 364 women over 55 years of age for the study, lead researcher Joanne Schneider, PhD, came to the realization that those who believed the most in the benefits of exercise were the ones who benefited the most physiologically and psychologically by exercising for longer periods of time and with more intensity.

#99 Change Your Destiny

There is a very famous quote from an unknown author that pretty much sums up the message of this chapter and ultimately this book:

> *"Watch your thoughts, for they become words. Watch your words, for they become actions. Watch your actions, for they become habits. Watch your habits, for they become character. Watch your character, for it becomes your destiny."*

So, in case you haven't gotten it by now, unless you believe 100 percent—within your soul—that you are ready to make a change in your life (i.e., lose the excess fat), no matter what you do, you will be destined for failure time and time again. But once you truly believe that change is not only possible but merely a matter of time, your personality and behaviors will guide you to your ultimate destiny—in this case, the new leaner, more energetic You!

"Within you right now is the power to do things you never dreamed possible. This power becomes available to you just as you can change your beliefs." —Author Unknown

BONUS CHAPTER

LOSING FAT 4 LIFE EATING PRINCIPLES

I have never known anyone to get excited about starting a diet, which is exactly why **Losing Fat 4 Life** is about embracing the proper foods at the proper times of the day—NOT ABOUT COUNTING CALORIES! That's right, I am not a believer in calorie counting for the reason, this method of fat loss is very rarely if ever successful—especially in the long term.

You'll notice I used the term "fat loss" as opposed to "weight loss" and this is because calorie counting does nothing to ensure that you will hold onto valuable muscle tissue. In fact, as I pointed out, very often fad diets (i.e., low calorie or low-fat diets) cause you to lose just as much muscle as fat, which is not smart if you truly want to lose fat for life. **Losing Fat 4 Life** contains strategies you can follow for life (and here you thought the name was just another marketing gimmick!). Aside from all this, who wants to count every calorie, every day, for the rest of their lives anyway?

The reason I am so convinced that the principles outlined in **Losing Fat 4 Life** will help you achieve your optimal metabolism, is because these very principles have been used—with much success—for over ten years by tens of thousands of people all over the world. My first book, <u>Fat Wars 45 Days to Transform Your Body</u>, changed thousands of people's lives for the better. Fat loss is my first love (aside from my family of course) and I have taken fat loss to a whole new understanding (physiologically and physiologically speaking) in my upcoming book <u>Sell You Lite</u> (Spring 2011 release).

Losing Fat 4 Life eating principles are based upon portion control for your individual uniqueness. After following the eating plan for a relatively short period of time, your body will adjust its metabolism to allowing its own fat stores to become the preferred source of fuel for your body.

It is important to note that **Losing Fat 4 Life** is about *eating*, *enjoying* and *embracing* nutrient dense foods rather than *avoiding* them. Now there's a concept you can sink your teeth into! It is also important to understand that **Losing Fat 4 Life** is designed to educate you on how to eat to achieve and then maintain a healthy metabolism for the rest of your life. This in no way means that you can never reward yourself with so-called "fun foods" (and you know what these are), but the goal is to establish a healthy metabolism first (which can take a few months) before you start including "fun foods" in your diet.

The **Losing Fat 4 Life** principles consist of consuming proper nutrition (including effective supplementation) at regular intervals throughout the day. This is why I advocate eating three solid meals and consuming two high quality protein shakes—preferable from High-Alpha Whey Protein—per day. These meals are to be consumed every three to four hours—for optimal metabolic effect. By consuming smaller portions of nutrient dense foods throughout the day, your body is able to balance blood sugar chemistry, keep insulin levels in check and reduce cravings more effectively.

To function optimally, the human body requires essential nutrients—which are nutrients that your body cannot manufacture on its own. These are: water, minerals, vitamins, carbohydrates, fats and proteins.

- **Water** regulates all functions of the body (see Chapter 6).

- **Minerals** regulate processes within the body that help generate enzymes, hormones, skeletal bones, muscle, teeth and fluids (visit www.LeafSource.com for one of the best natural mineral formulas available today).

- **Vitamins** are found in fruits, vegetables, meats, and whole grains. Vitamins provide energy to the body and are needed in small amounts to assist the chemical reactions within our cells.

- **Proteins** help stabilize blood sugar, promote cell growth and repair, assist hormone production, enzyme production (digestive and metabolic), neurotransmitter production, cell metabolism, body fluid balancing, maintenance of the immune system and are essential to a healthy metabolism (see Chapter 7).

- **Carbohydrates** (only the low glycemic/non-processed variety) ensure energy production, thyroid conversion, and muscular repair and help maintain a proper balance of insulin to glucagon—to ensure effective fat burning (see Chapter 8).

- **Fats** (as in essential fatty acids— EFA's and monounsaturated fats) EFA's are essential to produce energy, construct cellular membranes, help detoxify the body, regulate cell traffic (keeping viruses and germs out—keeping cell proteins, organelles, enzymes and genetic material in), maintain healthy insulin functions, form red blood cells, lubricate our joints, and help us maintain an optimal metabolism. Good fats also ensure that we burn fat by increasing the amount of oxygen utilized by the cells to produce energy (see Chapter 9).

Constructing Your Meals

When planning a **Losing Fat 4 Life** friendly meal, it is important to include all essential nutrients. We all know how to find water, but what about the rest of these nutrients? Your vitamins and minerals should come primarily from fruits and vegetables (and supplementation is also wise, if the minerals are in a natural organic form, as found in LeafSource); however, it is important to note that conventionally grown foods can contain up to 90 percent less minerals than their organic counterparts.

The following is a quick overview as to which foods fall under the categories of **protein, carbohydrates** and **fats**.

Foods that contain Protein:

- Fish—salmon, cod, tuna, bass, halibut, snapper, swordfish, trout, haddock, sole
- Seafood—shrimp, scallops, lobster, crab, clams, oysters, mussels
- Poultry—free range: chicken breast, turkey breast, duck, ostrich, goose, quail
- Meat—game meats, tenderloin

- Eggs—organic and free run
- Milk products (these are your best choices)—plain organic yogurt, cottage cheese
- Protein formulas—whey protein (preferably High-Alpha Whey Protein), hemp, sprouted brown rice and Moringa.

Foods that contain healthy Carbohydrates:

- Fruits (preferably berries), vegetables (all non-starchy), nuts, legumes

Foods that contain Healthy fats:

- **Omega-3 fats:** flax, flaxseed oil, pumpkin seeds, walnuts, brazil nuts, hemp oil, cold water fish, krill, fortified egg yolks.
- **Omega-6 fats:** sunflower, safflower, sesame, corn, primrose, borage, blackcurrant seed oil, milk, egg yolks, warm-water fish, olive oil and avocados.

The Best Fats and Oils for Cooking

When cooking with these oils—cook over low to medium temperatures only):

- Olive Oil (extra virgin-cold pressed)
- Coconut Oil
- Walnut Oil
- Avocado Oil
- Butter

Measuring Your Protein Portion

When it comes to constructing a properly designed **Losing Fat 4 Life** meal, you should always start by fulfilling your protein needs. To do this, your protein choice should be the approximate <u>size</u> and <u>thickness of your palm</u>, which should equate to approximately **3-4oz. for a woman** and **4-6oz. for a man**.

Healthy Eggs

I recommend free range, organic omega-3 eggs for a couple of reasons. Free-range chickens are just that—free to roam and feed off the land as chickens were intended to do—and happy chickens usually equate to healthy chickens. As well, when chickens are raised on feed that is fortified with omega-3 fats, their eggs contain elevated levels of these beneficial fats—which as you will recall are not as abundant in our diet as their omega-6 counterparts.

Adding Your Carbohydrates and Healthy Fat Portions

Once you have your selected choice of protein, fill the rest of your plate with fibrous vegetables (which come from the recommended carbohydrate choices). Now this does not mean that you have to have salad every single night—your vegetables can be steamed, broiled, baked, or poached.

For the healthy fat portion of your **Losing Fat 4 Life** meals, use the healthy fat recommendations as salad dressings or vegetable toppings such as seeds and nuts.

Nuts and Seeds

All nuts and seeds must be fresh, unsalted, un-roasted and blanched (if the nut has a skin)—your best bet being raw.

Almonds	10 (average serving)
Cashews	9 (average serving)
Pecans	8 (average serving)
Pumpkin seeds	20 (average serving)
Pistachios	22 (average serving)
Walnuts	7 (average serving)
Sunflower seeds	25 (average serving)

Organic Is Always Best

Organic is always your best bet if given the option. Organic foods supply an enhanced nutritional value to your body's structure and are similar to the foods our ancestors ate. Organic foods are also free from unnecessary chemicals, preservatives, contaminants, and other harmful substances, such as pesticides, herbicides and fungicides. According to the Journal of Applied Nutrition, the majority of organic fruits, vegetables and grains have 90 percent more minerals than conventionally grown food.

The Problem with Grains

When it comes to grains, it is important to note that many grains cause a rapid rise in your insulin response—which places your body in a fat-storing mode by elevating insulin and the powerful fat-storage enzyme LPL. Aside from this, many people have a difficult time digesting gluten, which is the protein found in grains. According to the book Dangerous Grains, gluten intolerance does not just affect people with Celiac Disease (CD)—an allergic reaction to the grain found primarily in rye, oats and barley—but a great percentage of our population. In fact, the authors suggest that CD should actually be renamed "gluten sensitivity."

Sweeteners

There are many different artificial sweeteners on the market and it is in your best interest to familiarize yourself with the pros and cons of each of these. I am not a proponent of any artificial sweetener available today as these were never around as our intricate biochemistry was evolving and therefore may present problems to our bodies. The only natural sweeteners I presently advocate are *Stevia* and *Xylitol*, as these are both 100 percent natural and do not seem to negatively affect metabolism.

Processed Foods

I highly recommend avoiding *all* processed foods like the plague! These foods do nothing but strip the body of its own nutrient supplies and in the process elevate insulin levels, which ultimately make it next to impossible to use fat as energy.

Beware of Fructose

Although fructose is considered a natural sugar (and it is in fruit), often when it is added to foods and beverages—especially as high-fructose corn syrup—it can greatly enhance our ability to store fat and decrease metabolism. According to the research of Richard Johnson, MD, chief of the division of kidney disease and hypertension at the University of Colorado and one of the world's leading experts in this area, excess fructose consumption can lead to high blood pressure, obesity, and diabetes. Fruit juices contain exceptionally high levels of concentrated fructose—yes, even the "so-called" 100 percent natural juices. So beware!

Trans Fats

I highly recommend avoiding foods containing trans fats as they have been found to raise LDL cholesterol levels which is a major cause of heart disease. 40 percent of daily trans fat intake among North Americans comes from cakes, cookies, crackers, pies, bread and the like.

Out on the Town

Looking for the keys to eating out and being sociable without blowing everything you worked so hard for? Your success at **Losing Fat 4 Life** is largely determined by your lifestyle and dietary choices. In fact, every time you sit down to eat you are either moving one step closer to a fat burning metabolism—or one step closer to a fat storing one. Each and every day, and perhaps each hour, you are in a position to make a choice that advances your goals or sets them back.

Since it has taken most of us many years to transform into the shape and health we are presently experiencing, we cannot expect positive transformation overnight. One fat-promoting meal can easily turn into a second and so on, just as one day of lethargy can turn into a second and so on. We all have choices. Unfortunately, too many of us take the easy road and end up breaking down long before we reach the end.

It is not always easy to make the right choices, but the bottom line is we all have to live with the choices we make. Some of the hardest choices come in the form of *what* and *when* to eat when we are out for dinner or out on the road. Far too often we make food choices unconsciously in an effort to satisfy a need that is not tangible at the time. We need to be pre-emptive and make sure we plan for behaviors and situations, so we are always one step ahead.

Part of a winning approach is to anticipate the situations that will trigger old behaviors of poor eating habits. To help you avoid defeating behaviors, I will provide you with scenarios that suggest how to stay on the **Losing Fat 4 Life** road when eating out, during social situations and on the road.

Restaurant Eating

In spite of our good intentions to make healthful meals, our lives are filled with competing interests that draw us to making convenient choices. When eating out either at a trendy restaurant or fast-food outlet, consider these strategies:

- When you have a choice, choose a restaurant that provides a varied menu. Stay away from menus that do not allow you to make healthy choices. Some examples include hamburger joints, fish-and-chip restaurants, fried-chicken outlets and barbecued-rib restaurants.
- While at the restaurant, be strategic and choose foods that are wholesome instead of

processed. These unprocessed foods will not only provide you with the greatest amount of nutrients but also keep you full longer.

- Ask yourself questions when you are making a food choice at a restaurant. How much unhealthy fat does the food have? Does it contain good fats or bad ones? Fats provide the most calories for the lowest amount of nutrients. This is an important area to consider when you decide how much and what type of fat you will consume.

- When you sit down at a restaurant, sometimes a basket of bread gets brought to the table. It is always best to ask the waiter *not* to serve the bread at your table and avoid the temptation altogether. It is extremely rare to find a restaurant that serves healthful, stone-ground or sprouted-grain breads, so it is best to just say no! Eating the bread will stimulate the fat-storing high-insulin response, add calories to your meal and provide you with very little nutrient density. If you are in a situation where others at your table want bread, do your very best to avoid eating it.

- Make sure you choose a main dish that is not starch-based. Choose meals that are high in protein and low in starchy carbohydrates. Most restaurants are very accommodating, so don't be afraid to ask your waiter for options.

- Make sure to include a good portion of fibrous mixed vegetables with your protein source. For instance, if you are ordering steak, chicken or fish, try to forgo the baked potato or rice pilaf and instead opt for a nice serving of veggies or a big salad.

Here are a few simple suggestions that will help you construct a healthier meal at any restaurant:

- Ask for dressings and sauces on the side.
- Opt for fruit and/or vegetable-based sauces rather than creamy sauces.
- Choose meals that are poached, steamed, broiled, or baked, but never fried.
- Choose fruit or yogurt-based desserts. Have the occasional dark chocolate treat, but make that treat infrequent and small.

Don't Be Fooled Again

Don't be fooled into the belief that beverages don't contain calories just because they don't contain fat. Alcoholic beverages can contain an enormous number of sugars and calories and make you feel hungry rather than provide you with valuable nutrients. Always choose water as your beverage of choice at a restaurant and go for the glass of red wine once in a while. After all, you are human.

Foods that contain more fibers tend to fill you up and control the release of your fat-storing hormone, insulin. Therefore,

- Avoid refined rice and any white-flour products, including pasta.
- Go for large amounts and a wide variety of vegetables. If necessary, ask for a larger portion of your favorite vegetables (or a big salad).
- Remember to ask for steamed, broiled, baked, or poached vegetables that are not lathered in butter but lightly coated with olive oil.

The Following are My 9 Losing Fat 4 Life Eating Tips

1. Consume five mini meals per day (three solid—two protein shakes).
2. Make sure to eat every three to four hours in order to maintain blood sugar levels.
3. Include high quality protein in each and every meal—making sure to individualize your protein portion (see *Measuring your protein portion* in the Bonus Chapter).
4. Drink plenty of water. A good rule of thumb is to consume one

liter of water for every 50 pounds of bodyweight and don't forget to include 8 oz. of filtered water approximately 20 minutes prior to each meal in order to curb your appetite.

5. Watch your consumption of fruit juices, as they often contain too much fructose and completely avoid fruit drinks with added sugars.

6. Never overeat.

7. Eat slowly and stop when you are hungry.

8. Don't consume carbs past 6:00 PM.

9. Always leave at least two hours between your last meal and bedtime.

ABOUT

THE

AUTHOR

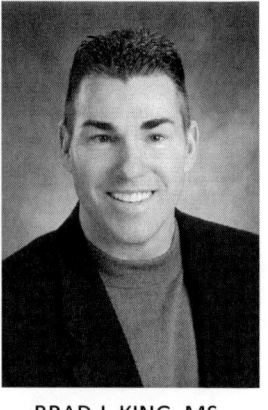

BRAD J. KING, MS, MFS

Brad has been referred to as one of the most influential health mentors of our time and is widely recognized as one of the most sought after authorities on nutrition, obesity, longevity and men's health.

After losing both of his parents to cancer within a six month period fifteen years ago, he has since dedicated his life to encouraging people to take charge of their health. Brad believes...*It's not that you age... it is how you choose to age that matters.*

Brad is the author of 10 books including the international best seller, <u>Fat Wars 45 Days to Transform Your Body</u>, and the award winning <u>Beer Belly Blues: What Every Aging Man and the Women in His Life Need to Know</u>.

Aside from being an inductee into the prestigious *Canadian Sports Nutrition Hall of Fame*, he also sits on the board of directors for CHI—the premiere sports nutrition education center.

Brad formulates the highest quality nutritional supplements for the natural health industry and has won many gold medal awards over the years for these products. He receives testimonials on a daily basis from those whose lives he has changed.

Brad's depth of knowledge and sense of humor make him a popular interview and he has been featured on thousands of television and radio programs as well as both magazine and newspaper articles throughout North America as a leading health expert. Some of these shows include: The Today Show, Canada AM, Balance TV, Macleans, Oxygen, The National Post, Chatelaine and The Vancouver Sun.

You can listen to Brad live every week at noon Pacific/3pm Eastern on his radio show *Transforming Health with Brad King* at www.VoiceAmerica.com The Health and Wellness Channel.

Getting Started:

Your basic recommended supplementation is:

- **Ultimate Multi**—2-4 capsules/day with meals – up to 8 capsules (4 in the morning and 4 in the evening) can be taken if extremely active or under excess stress

- **Ultimate High-Alpha Whey Protein**—2 shakes/day

- **Ultimate Sleep**—2-3 capsules taken approximately one half hour before bed

If you want to ensure you are Losing Fat 4 Life, the additional supplementation is recommended:

- **FibreLean**—1 scoop 5 minutes prior to meals or in shakes

- **Ultimate Calorie Burn**—2 capsules first thing in the morning.

- **Ultimate Anti-Stress**—2 capsules once or twice day when needed

Gender Specific Losing Fat 4 Life recommended supplementation:

HER Losing Fat 4 Life:
- **Her Energy**—2 capsules twice daily with meals

HIS Losing Fat 4 Life:
- **His Energy**—2 capsules twice daily with meals

Ultimate AM/PM Fat Loss Program

24 hour fat loss, reduce abdominal fat, enhance metabolism, reduce cravings, improve sleep, increase energy

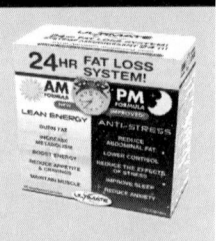

AM FORMULA: *Ultimate Lean Energy™*

Suggested Usage – AM Formula: Take 3 capsules of *Ultimate Lean Energy™* once or twice a day approximately 30 minutes before exercise or a meal. Best time to use is first thing in the morning and preferably on an empty stomach. It is not recommended to exceed 6 capsules a day.

PM FORMULA: *Ultimate Anti-Stress™ (see ingredients below)*

Suggested Usage – PM Formula: Take 2 capsules of *Ultimate Anti-Stress™* at bedtime.

Ultimate Anti-Stress™

Reduce abdominal fat, reduce cortisol levels, improve sleep, reduce fatigue, improve ability to deal with excess stress

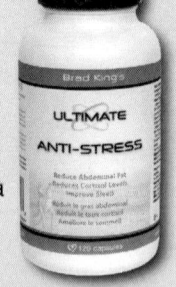

Each Capsule Contains: Sensoril™ Ashwagandha Extract (*Withania somnifera*) (root + leaf) (8% Withanolides), Valerian Extract (*Valeriana officinalis*) (root) (0.8%Valerenic Acid), Citrus Bioflavonoids, Lyophilized Adrenal Tissue, Quercetin, Rhodiola Extract (*Rhodiola rosea*) (root) (3.5% Rosavins), BioPerine® Black Pepper Extract (*Piper nigrum*) (fruit) (95% Piperine).

Suggested Usage: Take 2 capsules once or twice a day or as directed by a health care practitioner.

Ultimate Anti-Stress™ VEGAN

Reduce abdominal fat, reduce cortisol levels, improve sleep, reduce fatigue, improve ability to deal with excess stress

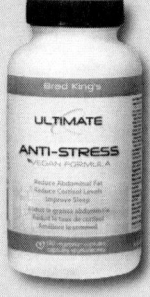

Each Capsule Contains: Lemon Balm Extract (*Melissa officinalis*) (leaf) (5% Rosemarinic acid), Citrus Bioflavonoids, Sensoril™ Ashwagandha Extract (*Withania somnifera*) (root and leaf) (8% Withanolides), Valerian Extract (*Valeriana officinalis*) (root) (0.8% Valerenic Acid), Quercetin, Rhodiola Extract (*Rhodiola rosea*) (root) (3.5% Rosavins), BioPerine® Black Pepper Extract (*Piper nigrum*) (fruit) (95% Piperine).

Suggested Usage: Take 2 capsules once or twice a day or as directed by a health care practitioner.

Ultimate Calm™

Anti-anxiety, supports relaxation, increases focus

Each Capsule Contains: 125 mg of Pharma GABA™ 80 complex providing the following: Pharma GABA 80 gamma-aminobutyric acid (natural source of glutamic acid).

Suggested Usage: Take 1-2 capsules 3 times daily or as directed by a health care practitioner.

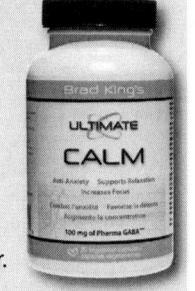

Ultimate Calorie Burn™

Burn calories, manage appetite and cravings, support healthy metabolism, reduce body fat, enhance mood, energy, endurance, stamina, mental acuity, focus and concentration

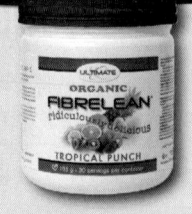

Each Capsule Contains: Chocamine™ Plus (*Theobroma cacao* extract blend with 8% caffeine), Capsimax™ (patented capsicum extract), BioPerine® Black Pepper Extract (*Piper nigrum*) (fruit) (Standardization 95% Piperine).

Note: Consult your health care practitioner if you take insulin or blood thinners. For best results, it is recommended to take small frequent breaks (i.e., a few days each month) from any product that contains caffeine.

Suggested Usage: Take 2 capsules 1–2 times daily before exercise or when maximal mental and physical energy demands are required. To ensure maximum effects and to avoid desensitization, do not take more than 5 times per week.

Ultimate FibreLean®

Promote bowel health, lower excess cholesterol, reduce excess body fat, reduce hunger

Formula: FibreLean 100% Organic Blend:
FOS, water soluable guar gum, flaxseed meal, a complex of fruit and vegetable fibre from the following sources: celery, apple, blueberry, blackberry and cranberry, natural flavour and silica.

Suggested Usage (Adults): For enhanced fat loss, take 1 scoop with a full 8oz. of filtered water approximately 20 minutes before a meal up to three times a day. You can also take one scoop at bedtime (along with full 8oz. of water). For general intestinal health, take 1-3 scoops 1-2 times daily with 8oz. of filtered water or mix with your protein shake twice daily (follow with an additional 8oz. of filtered water) or as directed by a health care practitioner. Please make sure to start out with lower amounts before going to three scoops.

FLAVOURS: Unflavoured, Black Cherry, Lemon Lime, Tropical Punch

Ultimate Her Energy™

Reduce abdominal fat, protect breast and uterine health, reduce PMS, reduce harmful estrogens

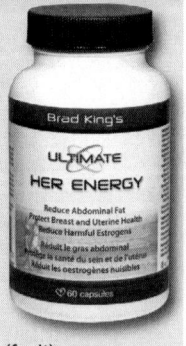

Each Capsule Contains: Citrus Bioflavonoids, Indole-3-Carbinol, d-Glucarate, Quercetin, Holy Basil (*Ocimum sanctum*) (leaf) (2% Ursolic Acid), Turmeric (*Curcuma longa*) (rhizome) (95% Curcumin), Milk Thistle Extract (*Silybum marianum*) (80% Silymarin), Broccoli (*Brassica oleracea*) (floret & stalk) (0.1% Sulforaphane), BioPerine® Black Pepper Extract (Piper nigrum) (fruit) (Standardization 95% piperine).

Suggested Usage: Take 2 capsules once or twice daily or as directed by a health care practitioner.

Ultimate Joint Relief™

Supports joint health, regulates inflammation, reduces pain sensivity, reduce muscle pain, reduce bone discomfort.

Each Capsule Contains: Juniper berry (*Juniperus communis*) 4:1 extract, Grape fruit (*Vitis vinifera*) 1:1 extract, Goldenrod flower (*Solidago Virgaures*) 4:1 extract, Dandelion leaf (*Taraxacum officinale*) 5.1 extract, Meadowsweet (*Filipendula ulmaria*) 4:1 extract, Willow bark (*Salix Alba*) 5:1 extract.

Suggested Usage: Take 2 capsules in the morning and if needed, another 2 capsules in the evening or as directed by a health care practitioner. Maintenance dose is 2 capsules in the morning on an empty stomach.

Ultimate Lean Energy™

Control appetite, enhance metabolism, reduce cravings, increase energy

Each Capsule Contains: Guarana Extract, Green Tea Extract 25:1 (*Camellia Sinensis*) (leaf), Yerba Maté Extract (*Ilex paraguariensis*) (leaf), (*Gymnema Sylvestre*) Extract 18:1 (75% Gymnemic Acids) (leaf), Cayenne (*Capsicum annum*) (fruit), Kelp Extract 4:1 (Ascophyllum nodosum) (whole plant), BioPerine Black Pepper Extract 1:5 (Piper nigrum) (fruit (Standardization 95% Piperine).

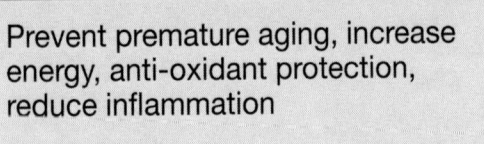

Caution is advised when taking prescription drugs that lower blood sugar levels. Patients taking oral drugs for diabetes or using insulin should be monitored closely by their health care provider while using this formula due to the gymnemic acids. Dosing adjustments may be necessary. Caution is advised when taking anticoagulants (blood thinners) or antiplatelet drugs and when using drugs to treat asthma, high blood pressure or glaucoma; or when taking drugs that increase heart rate or heart function.

Suggested Usage: The best time to use Lean Energy™ is first thing in the morning, preferably before a workout on an empty stomach and again in the later afternoon before a meal. Take 3 capsules once or twice a day approximately 30 minutes before exercise or a meal. It is not recommended to exceed 6 capsules a day.

Ultimate Longevity™

Prevent premature aging, increase energy, anti-oxidant protection, reduce inflammation

Each Capsule Contains: High ORAC Value Fruit Blend (Proprietary Ultra blend of the following: pomegranate, apple, elderberry, rosemary, white tea, blueberry, black current, raspberry), L-Carnosine, Ginger Extract 1:4 (Zingiber officinale) (root), Thyme Extract 1:4 (Thymus vulgaris) (leaf), L-Glutathione (GSH), Rosemary Extract 1:10 (Rosmarinus officinalis) (leaf) (6% Carnosic Acid), Pepper Extract (Piper nigrum) (fruit) (95% Piperin).

Suggested Usage: Take 1 capsule daily (preferably on an empty stomach) or as directed by a health care practitioner.

Maca

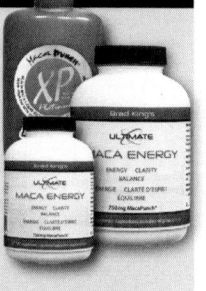

Reduce stress, improve mental clarity and memory, increase stamina, slow biological aging, improve libido, fight osteoporosis, relieve headaches, support balanced hormones, enhance immune system, increase energy

LIQUID EXTRACT: Each teaspoon contains: 100% fair-trade certified organic Black Maca Root, Water, Alcohol and Cellulose Gum.
Suggested Usage: Take it straight or mixed with your favourite drink or food 1-3 times daily.

POWDER: Each teaspoon contains: 100% fair-trade certified organic Gelatinized Maca Powder: 100% Maca roots.
Suggested Usage: Simply mix one or more teaspoons with your favourite drink or food 1-3 times daily.

CAPSULES: Each capsule contains: Organic Gelatinized Maca Powder.
Suggested Usage: 2-4 capsules a day or as directed by a health care practitioner.

Ultimate Migraine & Headache Relief™

Reduce pain signals, regulates brain inflammation, fast acting

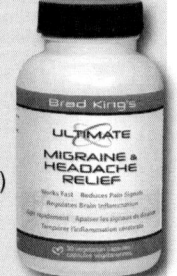

Each Capsule Contains: Juniper berry (*Juniperus communis*) 4:1 extract, Grape fruit (*Vitis vinifera*) 1:1 extract, Goldenrod flower (*Solidago Virgaures*) 4:1 extract, Dandelion leaf (*Taraxacum officinale*) 5.1 extract, Meadowsweet (*Filipendula ulmaria*) 4:1 extract, Willow bark (*Salix Alba*) 5:1 extract.

Suggested Usage: Take 2 capsules at the first sign of migraine once or twice daily or as directed by a health care practitioner. Maintenance dose is 2 capsules in the morning on an empty stomach.

Ultimate Multi™

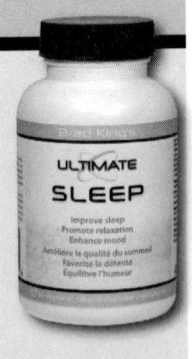

Increase energy, support metabolism, maintain healthy cardiovascular and nervous systems, enhance immunity, improve skin, hair and nails

Each Capsule Contains: Vitamin A (palmitate), Beta-carotene (*D. Salina*), Vitamin D3 (cholecalciferol), Vitamin E (mixed tocopherols), Vitamin C (calcium ascorbate), Calcium (citrate), Acerola Juice Powder, Ascorbyl Palmitate, Vitamin B1 (thiamine HCl), Vitamin B2 (riboflavin/ribof avin-5-phosphate), Vitamin B3 (inositol hexanicotinate), Vitamin B3 (niacinamide), Pantothenic Acid (calcium-d-pantothenate), Vitamin B5 (pantethine), Vitamin B6 (pyridoxine HCl/pyridoxyl-5-phosphate), Folic Acid 10%, Biotin, Vitamin B12 (methylcobalamin), Choline (citrate), Inositol, Magnesium (chelate), Potassium (citrate), Zinc (citrate), Manganese (citrate), Copper (gluconate), Iodine (potassium iodide), Selenium (selenomethionine), Chromium (Chromium454), Vanadium (picolinate), Molybdenum (citrate), Boron (FruiteX-B®), Silicon (bamboo leaf extract), Trimethylglycine, Citrus Bioflavonoids Powder, R - Alpha - Lipoic Acid, Bioperine® Black Pepper Extract (*Piper nigrum*) (fruit) (95% Piperin), Lutein Vg.

Suggested Usage: Take 2 to 4 capsules daily up to 8 capsules for maximum performance or as directed by a health care practitioner.

Ultimate Sleep™

Improve sleep, promote relaxation, enhance mood

Each Capsule Contains: 5-Hydroxytryptophan (Griffonia simplicifolia), Pumpkin seed extract, L-Lysine, Niacinamide, Melatonin, Jujube (Ziziphus jujuba) fruit extract (4:1), L-Theanine.

Suggested Usage: Take 2 to 3 capsules all at once before bedtime or as recommended by a health care practitioner.

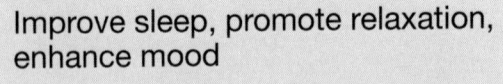

Ultimate Proteins

Ultimate High Alpha Whey Protein™

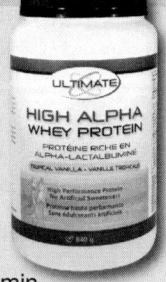

Lose fat, stop cravings, improve immune function, improve sleep, reduce stress, enhance hair, skin and nails; build and repair muscle; build, repair and replace body cells, enhance serotonin

Whey Protein Microfractions: 33% Alpha lactalbumin, 34-38% Beta-lactoglobulin, 19-22% Glycomacropeptides, 0.8-1.6% Albumin, 1% Lactoferrin, 0.8-2.4% Immunoglobulins

Suggested Usage: Mix an Ultimate Protein shake anytime you require a high source of protein. Mix 2 scoops (33g) in 250mL of water or juice.

Ultimate ISO Energy Whey Protein™

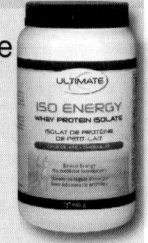

Lose fat, stop cravings, improve immune function, improve sleep, provide energy, enhance skin and nails; build and repair muscle, skin and bones; build, repair and replace body cells; regulate metabolic process

Whey Protein Microfractions: 14-18% Alpha lactalbumin, 43-48% Beta-lactoglobulin, 24-28% Glycomacropeptides, 1-2% Albumin, 1% Lactoferrin, 1-3% Immunoglobulins

Suggested Usage: Mix an Ultimate Protein shake anytime you require a high source of protein. Mix 2 scoops (36.7g) in 250mL of water or juice.

Ultimate Starch and Fat Blocker™

Prevent your body from storing over 50% of calories from most starches, block uptake of approximately 30% of calories from fat, prevent fat and excess sugars from entering the blood stream, regulate appetite

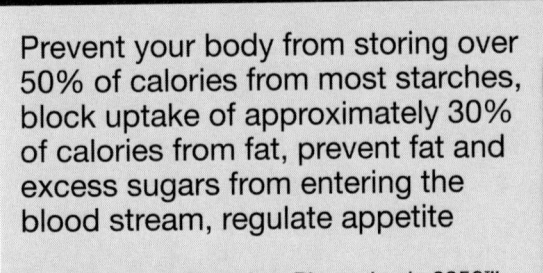

Each Capsule Contains: Phaseolamin 2250™ (Phase 2™) (Phaseolus vulgaris) (dried bean extract), (Opuntia ficus-indica), Gymnema Extract (Gymnema Syvestris) (leaf) (75% Gymnemic Acids), Green Tea Extract (Camellia sinensis) (80% Polyphenols) (leaf). Bioperine® Black Pepper Extract (Piper nigrum) (fruit) (Standardization 95% Piperine).

Caution is advised if on prescription medications unless under the supervision of a health care practitioner.

Suggested Usage: Take 3 capsules at the beginning of a high starch and/or high fat meal or as directed by a health care practitioner. Not to be used to maintain a poor diet.

Beer Belly Blues

In *Beer Belly Blues*, nutritional researcher and bestselling author Brad King uses humorous anecdotes as well as concise layman's prose to explain the complex underlying cause of age-related changes in men, and shows us how, when armed with knowledge and an enlightened strategy, we can safely recapture the energy and even the body of our youth.

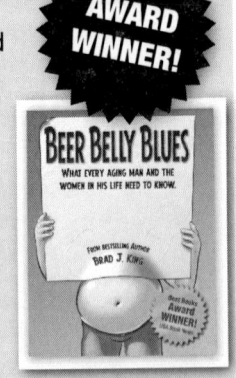

ISBN: 978-0-9810642-0-8

MEN'S HEALTH

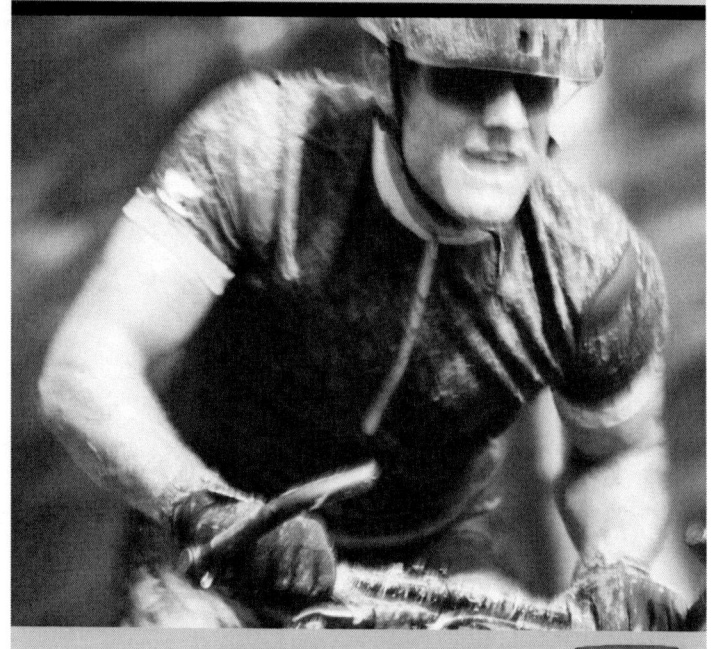

Ultimate Libido™

Enhance libido, boost desire and performance, increase the body's natural production of testosterone, maintain and build muscle tissue, enhance orgasm intensity and duration.

Each Capsule Contains: Tongkat Ali 100:1 Extract (*Eurycoma longifolia*) (root), Epimedium 4:1 Extract (*Epimedium grandiflorum*) (10% flavones) (stem and leaf), Damiana (*Turnera diffusa*) Powder (leaf), Zinc (Zinc Aminomin™), Niacin, Bioperine® Black Pepper Extract (Piper nigrum) (fruit) (Standardization 95% Piperine).

Suggested Usage: Take 3 capsules in the morning with or without food and another 3 approximately 1 hour prior to sexual activity or as directed by a health care practitioner. *Note: May cause male reproductive organ size increases (with higher doses).*

Ultimate Male Energy™

Enhance libido, increase testosterone, reduce abdominal fat, reduce harmful estrogens, maintain prostate health

Each Capsule Contains: Citrus Bioflavonoids, Chrysin (*Passiflora caerulea*) (flower), Turmeric (*Curcuma longa*) (rhizome) (95% Curcumin), Quercetin, Indole-3-Carbinol, Holy Basil (*Ocimum sanctum*) (leaf) (2% Ursolic acid), Nettle Extract 10:1 (*Urtica dioica*) (root), Broccoli (*Brassica oleracea*) (floret & stalk) (0.1% Sulforaphane), BioPerine® Black Pepper Extract (Piper nigrum) (fruit) (Standardization 95% piperine).

Suggested Usage: Take 2-4 capsules once or twice a day or as directed by a health care practitioner.

Ultimate Prostate™

Lower PSA levels, prevent prostate enlargement, reduce prostate inflammation, reduce urinary urgency and frequency, support prostate health, support healthy sexual function

Each Capsule Contains: Vegapure® FS Phytosterols (45% Beta Sitosterol), Nettle (*Urtica dioica*) Powdered Extract 10:1 (root), Flower Pollen (*Secale cereale*) Extract 20:1 (pollen), Pygeum Africanum (*Prunus africana*) Powdered Extract 15:1 (12% phytosterols) (bark), Indole-3 Carbinol, Broccoli (*Brassica oleracea*) Powdered Extract 15:1 (0.1% Sulforaphane) (floret and stalk), Lycopene [from 200mg of Lycomato® Tomato (Lycopersicon esculentum) (fruit)], Zinc (from Zinc Aminomin™), BioPerine® Black Pepper Extract (Piper nigrum) (fruit) (Standardization 95% piperine), Rosemary (*Rosmarinus officinalis*) Powdered Extract (6% carnosic acid) (leaf), Selenium (from Selenomethionine), Vitamin D3 (Cholecalciferol).

Suggested Usage: Take 3 capsules daily, with or without food or as directed by a health care practitioner.

Additional Titles in The 99 Series®

99 Things You Wish You Knew Before...
Facing Life's Challenges
Filling Out Your Hoops Bracket
Going Into Debt
Going Into Sales
Ignoring the Green Revolution
Landing Your Dream Job
Losing Fat 4 Life
Making It BIG In Media
Marketing On the Internet
Taking Center Stage

99 Things Women Wish They Knew Before...
Dating After 40, 50, and YES, 60!
Getting Behind the Wheel of Their Dream Job
Getting Fit Without Hitting the Gym
Entering the World of Internet Dating
Falling In Love
Hitting Retirement
Starting Their Own Business

99 Things Teens Wish They Knew Before Turning 16

99 Things Parents Wish They Knew Before Having "THE" Talk

99 Things Brides Wish They Knew Before Planning Their Wedding

www.99-Series.com